Math Basics for the Healthcare Professional

Math Basics for the Healthcare Professional
Second Edition

Michele Benjamin Lesmeister, MA

Renton Technical College

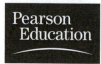

Pearson
Education

Upper Saddle River, New Jersey 07458

Library of Congress Cataloging-in-Publication Data

Benjamin-Lesmeister, Michele.
   Math basics for the healthcare professional /
Michele Benjamin Lesmeister.-- 2nd ed.
      p. cm.
Includes index.
  ISBN 0-13-113372-1
 1. Medicine--Mathematics. 2. Mathematics. 3. Medical sciences. I. Title.

R853.M3B46 2004
510--dc22   2003022459

Notice: The author and publisher of this volume have taken care that the information and technical recommendations contained herein are based on research and expert consultation, and are accurate and compatible with the standards generally accepted at the time of publication. Nevertheless, as new information becomes available, changes in clinical and technical practices become necessary. The reader is advised to carefully consult manufacturer's instructions and information material for all supplies and equipment before use, and to consult with a healthcare professional as necessary. This advise is especially important when using new supplies or equipment for clinical purposes. The author and publisher disclaim all responsibility for any liability, loss, injury, or damage incurred as a consequence, directly or indirectly, of the use and application of any of the contents of this volume.

Publisher: Julie Levin Alexander
Assistant to Publisher: Regina Bruno
Acquisitions Editor: Mark Cohen
Associate Editor: Melissa Kerian
Editorial Assistant: Mary Ellen Ruitenberg
Marketing Manager: Nicole Benson
Product Information Manager: Rachele Strober
Director of Production and Manufacturing: Bruce Johnson
Managing Production Editor: Patrick Walsh
Production Liaison: Danielle Newhouse

Production Editor: Patty Donovan, Pine Tree Composition
Manufacturing Manager: Ilene Sanford
Manufacturing Buyer: Pat Brown
Design Director: Cheryl Asherman
Design Coordinator: Maria Guglielmo Walsh
Cover Designer: Amy Rosen
Composition: Pine Tree Composition, Inc.
Printing and Binding: Banta Book Group
Cover Printer: Phoenix Color Corp.

Pearson Education, Ltd., *London*
Pearson Education Australia Pty. Limited, *Sydney*
Pearson Education Singapore Pte. Ltd.
Pearson Education North Asia Ltd., *Hong Kong*
Pearson Education Canada, Ltd., *Toronto*
Pearson Educación de Mexico, S.A. de C.V.
Pearson Education—Japan, *Tokyo*
Pearson Education Malaysia, Pte. Ltd.
Pearson Education, Upper Saddle River, New Jersey

10 9 8 7 6 5 4 3 2 1
ISBN 0-13-113372-1

Contents

Unit 4
Decimals   56

Preface for Educators and Learners

Math Basics for the Healthcare Professional was written to serve a large population of learners preparing for careers within health occupations as well as those working toward employment upgrades in the field. Suggested specific applications of this workbook are high school vocational programs; adult education programs that prepare students for health fields; self-study by individuals preparing for workplace transitions, upgrades, or changes; pre-nursing studies; and in-house or on-the-job training programs and general brush-up for work in the health care professions. The workbook was designed with student success in mind.

The workbook focuses on the needs of adult learners and features the following learner-based tools for success:

- sequential skill building on basic skills
- ties to the application of the skill with each math skill
- mnemonic devices to build memory of the basic skills
- a variety of practice opportunities with occupation-based examples and problems
- mixed applications which build on the basic skills and promote critical thinking
- self-tests to promote confidence and skill-building
- white spaces for thinking and working through the problems.

These materials have been successfully applied to help students prepare for a wide variety of health care training fields at a technical college. The student feedback and input has played a prominent role in the design and sequencing of the material, the methods of teaching, and presenting to new students. Thus, the organization of the text is central to the student's success. The students who have worked through these materials have been successful in their vocational training and workplace upgrading because they have reached a mastery level in the fundamental concepts; they are ready for the additional concepts and applications of their specific training areas.

The author has nearly 20 years of experience teaching a wide variety of adults: including second-language learners, industry experts, college preparatory students, public agency personnel, and other faculty. She embraces the attitude that all students can learn math; furthermore, she believes that the student's success is often tied to the presentation of materials. Therefore, the colloquial quality of this text's explanation of math processes creates a can-do approach and image of math. In health care, math is a job skill, and in turn, this proficiency will promote more job opportunities.

The second edition of this work text provides a reorganization of the metric system unit so that it is placed with Roman numerals and the apothecary system in Unit 8. This fits into the dosage calculations and allows the student to use the metric system as part of the dosage calculation. This contextualization helps students appreciate the value of learning the metric system conversions. In addition, extra practice problems have been included in most units. The unit self-tests include 15 questions, providing more practice in self-assessment. This edition has provided the odd numbers answers in the key at the end of the work text.

The Instructor's Guide has reproducible tests that accompany the workbook as a ready test bank on which instructors can rely. The unit tests (two per unit) ask the student to perform math calculations similar to those in the units. These unit tests each require 25 answers; thus, the tests do not overwhelm the student, but promote self-reliance and confidence building in math.

Two final post-tests are included which asks students to supply a total of 50 answers.

Acknowledgments

I would like to thank the reviewers of this book for their suggestions, comments, and encouragement. Their encouragement and feedback are greatly appreciated. These reviewers include:

Terri Ann Calnan, PN
Instructor/Program Director, Medical Assistant Program
Renton Technical College
Renton, WA

Vincent Range, MAT
ATS Math Department
Jefferson College
Hillsboro, MO

Cynthia Smathers, RRT
Respiratory Program Director
PIMA Medical Institute, Mesa Campus
Mesa, AZ

Janice Vermiglio-Smith, RN, MS, PhD.
Professor
Central Arizona College
Chandler, AZ

Math Basics for the
Healthcare Professional

Unit 1

Health Occupations Matrix of Math Skills and Self-Assessment

Each health care field has its own emphasis and requirements for math skills. Many successful adults search out materials that serve their immediate learning needs because their studies are just one part of their busy day. This workbook has been designed to help you measure your readiness for additional math training in and for your specific field.

To assist individuals new to health occupations, a matrix of skills has been developed to answer the question: What math do I need to know to be a _____? Refer to the matrix to attain a general idea of the math skills necessary for your program preparation or workplace upgrade. These skills will form the core of your math abilities, and you will build on them in more specific ways within your specific field of study.

Once you understand what math skills are needed for your program success, you are ready to take the self-assessment. This tool is divided into categories that match the workbook's content to help you work independently or within a classroom, and it allows you to begin at your own comfort or skill level. The idea is to provide enough review and practice so that you are able to calculate the problems for your program accurately and efficiently. Use the scoring sheet to prepare an individualized study plan for yourself or as a sheet to refer to when these units are covered to ensure that you have mastered the material.

By completing this workbook, you will be ready for the specific math training that you will receive in your program of study or from the workplace.

A final word about calculators: Calculators are wonderful tools. However, at this time, calculator use may be limited to certain instances, and calculators may or may not be allowed on exams. For these reasons, mental math is a valuable skill to review. Put your calculator away as you work through these

Table 1–1   Matrix of Skills

	Certified Nursing Assistant	Hospital Nursing Assistant	Massage Therapist	Dental Assistant	Pharmacy Technician	Surgical Technologist	Medical Assistant	Licensed Practical Nurse	Registered Nurse	Your Program Choices		
Unit 1: Matrix of Skills and Self-Assessment	X	X	X	X	X	X	X	X	X			
Unit 2: Whole Number Review	X	X	X	X	X	X	X	X	X			
Unit 3: Fractions	X	X	X	X	X	X	X	X	X			
Unit 4: Decimals	X	X	X	X	X	X	X	X	X			
Unit 5: Ratio and Proportion	X	X	X	X	X	X	X	X	X			
Unit 6: Percents			X	X	X	X	X	X	X			
Unit 7: Combined Applications			X	X	X	X	X	X	X			
Unit 8: Dosage Calculations					X	X	X	X	X			
Practice Post-Test	X	X	X	X	X	X	X	X	X			

materials, and two things will result: your proficiency will increase, and your self-confidence will soar as you become an efficient math problem solver.

Health Occupations Math Skills Self-Assessment Score Sheet

Take the self-assessment that begins on page 4. Then develop an individualized plan of study by checking the problems missed on the self-assessment.

Unit 2: Whole Numbers

_____ **a.**   Addition

_____ **b.**   Subtraction

_____ **c.**   Multiplication

_____ **d.**   Multiplication Word Problem

_____ **e.**   Division

_____ **f.**   Rounding

_____ **g.**   Averages

Unit 3: Fractions

____ **a.** Addition

____ **b.** Subtraction

____ **c.** Multiplication

____ **d.** Multiplication Word Problem

____ **e.** Division

____ **f.-g.** Complex Fractions

Unit 4: Decimals

____ **a.** Rounding

____ **b.** Averages

____ **c.** Temperature Conversion

____ **d.** Ordering Decimals

____ **e.** Addition

____ **f.** Subtraction

____ **g.** Multiplication

____ **h.** Division

Unit 5: Ratio and Proportion

____ **a.** Ratio

____ **b.** Solving Simple Proportions

____ **c.-d.** Proportion with Complex Fractions

____ **e.** Proportion in Word Problems

Unit 6: Percents

____ **a.** Finding Simple Percent

____ **b.** Finding Complex Percent

Unit 7: Combined Applications

____ **a.** Converting among Systems

____ **b.** Standard and Metric Measurements

____ **c.** Applied Proportion

____ **d.-g.** Mixed Applications

Unit 8: Dosage Calculations

____ **a.** Metric Conversions

____ **b.** Roman Numerals

____ **c.** Apothecary Conversions

____ **d.** Dosage Formula

Health Occupations Math Skills Self-Assessment

Show all of your work clearly.

Unit 2: Whole Numbers
Compute each answer.

a. The nursing assistant counts the latex examining gloves in each examination room. Determine the total: Room A: 234; Room B: 189; Room C: 54; and Room D: 546.

b. $76,000 - 4,629$

c. 134×69

d. The licensed practical nurse is giving a patient 250 milligrams of a medication to a patient in Room 1208 three times a day. How many milligrams of the medication is the nurse giving the patient each day?

e. $26,325 \div 250$

f. Round each number to the designated place value.

2,387   to the nearest   tens   _____

4,492   to the nearest   hundreds _____

g. Find the average weekly earnings:

Bob: $300; Sylvia: $258; Sam: $197; Bart: $320; and Mickey: $465.

Unit 3: Fractions

Reduce to the lowest terms.

a. $4\frac{2}{3} + 5\frac{1}{24}$

b. $8\frac{1}{16} - 3\frac{1}{4}$

c. $5 \times 9\frac{2}{3}$

d. How many seconds are there in $10\frac{2}{3}$ minutes?

e. $27\frac{1}{2} \div 5\frac{1}{5}$

f. $\dfrac{1/250}{1/300}$

g. $\dfrac{3/4}{1/8}$

Unit 4. Decimals

a. Round each number to the designated place value.

17.86	to the nearest	tenth	_____
17.578		hundredth	_____
17.0589		thousandth	_____

b. Averages: Find the averages and round the answer as appropriate for the specific application.

_____ 79.8°F, 68.9°F, 101.1°F

_____ $17.95, $13.45, $27.05, $2.09, $9.99

c. Temperature Conversion:

58°F equals how many degrees Celsius? _____

Convert 38°C into degrees Fahrenheit. _____

d. Arrange in order from smallest to largest:

0.25, 0.125, 0.3, 0.009, 0.1909 _____

Compute each answer:

e. 15.24 + 0.63

f. 1020 − 250.8

g. A radiologic technician can purchase x-ray film at $78.76 for 20 exposures or $108.90 for 30 exposures. If both films are of equal quality, which is the better buy?

h. 4.68 ÷ 0.06

Unit 5: Ratio and Proportion

a. Provide an equivalent ratio for $\frac{1}{4}$.

Solve for X.

b. $\dfrac{8}{64} = \dfrac{15}{x}$

c. $\dfrac{\frac{1}{2}}{2} = \dfrac{5\frac{2}{3}}{x}$

   d. Grains $^1/_4$: 1 tablet = grains $^1/_8$: x tablets

   e. To mix plaster for a dental model, 45 milliliters of water to 100 grams of plaster is used. How many milliliters of water are required for 200 grams of plaster?

Unit 6: Percents

   a. Find 24% of 125.

   b. What is $87^1/_2$% of 156?

Unit 7: Combined Applications

   a. Convert between systems. Reduce to lowest terms.

Fractions	Decimals	Ratio	Percent
$^2/_5$	_____	_____	_____
_____	_____	_____	17%
_____	0.54	_____	_____
_____	_____	1:5	_____

Fill in the blanks.

   b. Standard measurement and metric conversions:

   2 tablespoons = _____ teaspoons

   8 pints = _____ quarts

   _____ ounces = 2 cups

   1 fluid ounce = _____ tablespoon(s)

   23.5 kilograms = _____ pounds

   c. If 9 ounces of homemade soup contain 125 calories, 19 grams of carbohydrates, 1,150 milligrams of sodium, 4 grams of fat and 420 milligrams of potassium, then:

How much potassium is in 6 ounces of soup? _____

How many grams of carbohydrates are there in 12 ounces of soup? _____

How many calories are available in one cup of soup? Round to the nearest whole number. _____

Solve for X.

d. $\dfrac{25\%}{1/3} = \dfrac{0.5}{x}$

e. $\dfrac{35}{125} \times 12.5$

f. $\dfrac{15\%}{1/4}$

g. $\dfrac{1}{100} \times 3.5$

Unit 8. Dosage Calculations

a. Metric System: Convert each of the following:

How many milligrams equal 1.85 grams? _____

0.56 milligrams equal how many micrograms? _____

2.3 meters equal how many centimeters? _____

13.625 kilograms = _____ grams

1 liter contains _____ milliliters

b. Roman Numerals: Provide the equivalent Roman and Arabic numerals:

XVIII = _____

109 = _____

DIL = _____

64 = _____

viss = _____

c. Make the following conversions:

$1\frac{1}{2}$ ounces = ____ milliliters

0.6 milligrams = grains ____

4 drams = ____ milliliters

grains $\frac{3}{4}$ = ____ milligrams

grains vi = ____ minims

d. Use the formula: $\dfrac{\text{Dosage}}{\text{Supply on hand}} \times \text{Quantity}$

Order: 0.125 milligrams
Supply: 0.25 milligrams of scored tablets

Give _____

Order: Grains $\frac{1}{8}$ pain medication
Supply: 7.5 milligram tablets

Give _____

Order: 0.15 micrograms
Supply: 0.3 milligrams of scored tablets

Give _____

Order: Grains $\frac{1}{6}$
Supply: Elixir 20 milligrams per 5 milliliters

Give _____

Order: 1.5 grams
Supply: 750 milligrams capsules

Give _____

Unit 2

Whole Number Review

Mathematics is a key skill of health care workers. As a health care worker, you know that accuracy is important. Being competent in whole number concepts and addition, subtraction, multiplication, and division will form the basis for successful computations on the job. These basic skills form the foundation for the other daily math functions you will use in the workplace.

> Approach math matter of factly; math is a job skill and a life skill.

Addition

Review   To add, line up the numbers in a vertical column and add to find the total. In addition problems, the total, or answer, is called the *sum*.

Practice   Find the sum of each problem.

1. $1 + 4 + 5 + 9 =$
2. $51 + 23 =$
3. $297 + 90 + 102 + 3 =$
4. $216 + 897 =$
5. $1,773 + 233 + 57 =$
6. $9 + 245 + 32 =$
7. $11 + 357 + 86 + 34 =$

8. 24,578 + 9,075 =

9. 443 + 2,087 + 134 =

10. 910 + 3 + 125 =

Applications Inventory is an important clerical function in the health care industry. Sometimes this work is done by supply technicians, clerks, nursing assistants, or other staff. Keeping accurate inventory reduces overstocking and helps avoid the problem of under stocking medical supplies.

1. Inventory is done monthly at the Golden Years Care Center. Find the sum for each category.

Category	Sum
a. Examination gloves: 31 + 88 + 47 + two boxes of 50	_____
b. Thermometer covers: 281 + 304 + 17 + 109	_____
c. Medicine cups: 313 + 245 + 106 + 500 + 12	_____
d. Boxes of disposable syringes (50 per box): 2 + 6 + 9 + 3	_____

2. Intake and output totals require addition skills. Unlike household measurements in cups, health care patient intake and output units are measured in cubic centimeters (cc). Intake includes oral ingestion of fluids and semi-liquid food, intravenous feedings, and tubal feedings.
   Find the intake totals.

Type of Intake	Cubic Centimeters	Sum
a. Oral	120, 210, 150, 240	_____
b. Intravenous	250, 500	_____
c. Blood	500	_____
d.	Total Intake	_____

   The intake sums would be charted in the patient's medical record.

3. Measuring output is important because it helps the health care worker ensure a patient's health and hydration. Output is measured in cubic centimeters. Output includes liquid bowel movements or diarrhea, urine, emesis (vomiting), and gastric drainage.

Type of Output	Cubic Centimeters	Sum
a. Diarrhea	100, 200	_____
b. Urine	330, 225, 105, 60	_____
c. Gastric Drainage	40, 35	_____
d. Blood/Emesis	110	_____
e.	Total Output	_____

4. Assuming that the patient is the same as in problems 2 and 3, has this patient had a greater intake or a greater output? _____

Subtraction

Review   To subtract, line up the numbers according to place value. Place value shows the ones, tens, hundreds, etc. columns. Start with the rightside of the math problem and work your way toward the left side, subtracting each column.

> Fewer errors occur if the subtraction problem is set up vertically. Rewrite the problems.

Example

$$89 - 31 = \underline{\hspace{1cm}} \qquad\qquad 475 - 34 = \underline{\hspace{1cm}}$$

$$
\begin{array}{r}
89 \\
-31 \\
\hline
58
\end{array}
\qquad\qquad
\begin{array}{r}
475 \\
-34 \\
\hline
441
\end{array}
$$

If a number cannot be subtracted from the number directly above it, borrow one from the number in the column to the left.

> Keep track of borrowing by marking through the column borrowed from and reducing the numbers involved by 1.

Example

$$
\begin{array}{r}
3\,{}^{7}8\,{}^{1}1 \\
- \;\; 65 \\
\hline
316
\end{array}
$$

Practice

1. $475 - 81 =$

2. $176 - 37 =$

3. $289 - 54 =$

4. $4{,}547 - 2{,}289 =$

5. $1{,}236 - 799 =$

6. $1{,}575 - 896 =$

7. $2{,}001 - 128 =$

8. $10{,}300 - 497 =$

9. $4{,}301 - 89 =$

10. $4{,}547 - 2{,}289 =$

Applications   Subtraction is used in inventory as well. Some applications are given below.

1. At the beginning of the month, a dental office started with 2,258 latex examination gloves. On the last working day of the month, 784 remained. How many gloves were used during the month?

2. Inventory of dental file labels is to be kept at 2,000. Paula's inventory indicates 579 on hand. How many labels does she need to order?

3. Labels come in boxes of 500. Use the answer from problem 2 to determine how many boxes of labels Paula should order to obtain the required 2,000 minimum inventory. Draw a sketch to help visualize this problem.

4. Patients see the dentist most during the summer months. Dr. Brown has a total of 13,576 patient files. If he sees 8,768 of these patients during the summer, how many remain to be contacted for an appointment?

Multiplication

Memorizing the multiplication tables is essential to solid mental math. If you have been calculator dependent or have forgotten some of the tables, practice memorizing the multiplication tables using the chart shown in Table 2–1.

Review To multiply, line up the numbers according to place value. By putting the largest number on top of the problem, you will avoid careless errors.

> **Avoid These Common Errors**
>
> Remember, you are multiplying, not adding.
>
> Remember to move the numbers from the second and succeeding lines over one column to the left—use a zero (0) to indicate these movements.

Table 2–1   Multiplication Table

X	1	2	3	4	5	6	7	8	9	10	11	12
1												
2												
3												
4												
5												
6												
7												
8												
9												
10												
11												
12												

$2 \times 14 = $ _____ $\rightarrow 14$
                             $\underline{\times \; 2}$
                               28

     178
$\underline{\times \quad 23}$
     534
   $\underline{3560}$
   $4,094$

Move the second line of numbers one place to the left. Adding a zero keeps your numbers aligned.

Practice

1. $\begin{array}{r} 12 \\ \underline{\times 8} \end{array}$ **4.** $\begin{array}{r} 70 \\ \underline{\times 9} \end{array}$ **7.** $\begin{array}{r} 512 \\ \underline{\times 24} \end{array}$ **10.** $\begin{array}{r} 803 \\ \underline{\times 17} \end{array}$

2. $\begin{array}{r} 82 \\ \underline{\times 13} \end{array}$ **5.** $\begin{array}{r} 1,020 \\ \underline{\times 98} \end{array}$ **8.** $\begin{array}{r} 927 \\ \underline{\times 35} \end{array}$ **11.** $\begin{array}{r} 346 \\ \underline{\times 12} \end{array}$

3. $\begin{array}{r} 1,306 \\ \underline{\times 18} \end{array}$ **6.** $\begin{array}{r} 189 \\ \underline{\times 27} \end{array}$ **9.** $\begin{array}{r} 5,791 \\ \underline{\times 16} \end{array}$ **12.** $\begin{array}{r} 9,004 \\ \underline{\times 73} \end{array}$

Applications

1. Last month a nurse worked fourteen 10-hour shifts and two 12-hour shifts. At $21 per hour, what was the nurse's hourly income before deductions?

2. Health care facilities monitor all medications taken by their patients. Assume that the same dosage is given each time the medication is dispensed. What is the total daily dosage of each medication received?

Total Medication Received

a. Patient Bao   50 milligrams   4 times a day   _____ milligrams

b. Patient Mary   25 milligrams   2 times a day   _____ milligrams

c. Patient Luke   125 micrograms   3 times a day   _____ micrograms

d. Patient Vang   375 micrograms   2 times a day   _____ micrograms

3. The radiology lab ordered 15 jackets for its staff. The jackets cost approximately $35 each. What is the estimated cost of this order?

Division

Review To divide whole numbers, determine: a) what number is being divided into smaller portions and b) the size of the portions.

Division can appear in three formats:

   a. $27 \div 3 =$

   b. Twenty-seven divided by three

   c. $3\overline{)27}$

Setting up the problem correctly will help ensure the correct answer.

Example

$$81 \quad \div \quad 3 = \underline{\hspace{1cm}}$$

$\quad\quad\;\uparrow \quad\quad\;\; \uparrow$

dividend divisor

means eighty-one divided by three or how many 3s are in 81.
The answer is the quotient.

$$
\begin{array}{r}
27 \leftarrow \text{quotient} \\
\text{divisor} \rightarrow 3\overline{)81} \leftarrow \text{dividend} \\
\underline{6} \\
21 \\
\underline{21} \\
0
\end{array}
$$

Practice the correct setup, but do not work the problems.

1. Divide 145 by 76

2. $1,209 \div 563$

3. Forty-nine divided by seventeen is what number?

4. What is $8,794 \div 42$?

5. A person works a total of 2,044 hours a year. How many days does the person work if he works 8 hours a day?

Follow the steps below to complete all of your whole number division problems:

Step 1: Underline the number of places that the divisor can go into, then put the number of times the divisor can go into the dividend on the quotient line. Place it directly above the underlined portion of the number. This keeps track of your process. Multiply the number by the divisor and place it below the underlined portion of the dividend. Then subtract the numbers.

$$\begin{array}{r} 1 \\ 34\overline{)5492} \\ -34 \\ \hline 20 \end{array}$$

Step 2: Bring down the next number of the dividend. Use an arrow to keep alignment and track of which numbers you have worked with. Then repeat step 1.

$$\begin{array}{r} 161 \\ 34\overline{)5492} \\ -34\downarrow \\ \hline 20 \end{array}$$

$$\begin{array}{r} 161 \text{ R } 18 \\ 34\overline{)5492} \\ -34\downarrow \\ \hline 209 \\ 204\downarrow \\ \hline 52 \\ 34 \\ \hline 18 \end{array}$$

Repeat steps 1 and 2 until all the numbers of the dividend have been used. The number remaining is called the remainder. Place it next to an "R" to the right of the quotient. In fractions, the remainder becomes a fraction; in whole numbers, it remains a whole number.

After bringing a number down from the dividend, a number must be placed in the quotient. Zeros may be used as place holders. Follow the division steps as shown above to solve the practice problems.

$$\begin{array}{r} 106 \text{ R } 41 \\ 75\overline{)7991} \\ -75\downarrow \\ \hline 49 \\ -0\downarrow \\ \hline 491 \\ -450 \\ \hline 41 \end{array}$$

Practice   1. $6\overline{)564}$ 5. $4\overline{)1{,}244}$ 9. $2\overline{)46{,}882}$

2. $3\overline{)5{,}736}$ 6. $53\overline{)5{,}088}$ 10. $18\overline{)12{,}564}$

3. $4\overline{)12{,}345}$ 7. $15\overline{)23{,}648}$ 11. $7\overline{)87{,}543}$

4. $956 \div 66 =$ 8. $1{,}254 \div 29 =$ 12. $74{,}943 \div 271 =$

Applications   1. Room rates vary by the services provided. At the local hospital, intensive care unit (ICU) rooms are $784 a day. Bob's overall room charge was $10,192. How many days was Bob in ICU?

2. Carbohydrates have 4 calories per gram. If a serving of soup has 248 calories of carbohydrates, how many grams of carbohydrate are in that serving of soup?

3. A medical assistant subscribes to 14 magazines for the office. If the total subscription bill is $294, what is the average cost of each magazine subscription?

4. A pharmacy technician receives a shipment of 302 boxes of acetaminophen. This shipment needs to be returned to the supplier because the expiration date on the medicine did not allow sufficient time to sell the medicine. If each case holds 36 individual boxes, how many cases must the pharmacy technician use to pack the medicine?

5. A surgical technologist made $39,744 last year. He is paid twice a month. What is the gross or total amount of each of his paychecks?

6. A licensed practical nurse gives 1,800 milligrams of a penicillin-type drug over a 36-hour time period. If the dosage occurs every 6 hours, how many milligrams are in each dose if each dose is the same amount?

7. Each gram of fat contains 9 calories. How many grams of fat are in 81 calories of fat in a piece of steak?

Rounding

Review Whole numbers have place values. The number 3,195 has four specific place values: $\dfrac{3, \quad 1 \quad 9 \quad 5}{\underset{\text{thousand}}{\uparrow} \quad \underset{\text{hundreds}}{\uparrow} \quad \underset{\text{tens}}{\uparrow} \quad \underset{\text{ones}}{\uparrow}}$ (three thousand one hundred ninety-five)

By using the place values in a number, we can round the number to a particular and specific place unit. Rounding is valuable because it helps to estimate supplies, inventory, and countable items to the nearest unit.

> Rounding is used when an exact number is not necessary, as in taking inventory and ordering: Round up to make a full case of a product when you are placing an order. If a full case has 36 boxes and you need to order 32 boxes, you will order 1 case or 36 boxes, so you've rounded up to the nearest case.

Rounding is accomplished in three steps.

Example Round 7,872 to the nearest hundred.

Step 1: Locate the hundreds place and underline it.

$$7,\underline{8}72$$

Step 2: Circle the number to the right of the underlined number.

$$7,8\,⑦2$$

Step 3: If the circled number is 5 or greater, add 1 to the underlined number and change the number(s) to the right of the underlined number to zero(s).

$$7,\ \underline{8}\ ⑦\ 2$$
$$\downarrow\ \downarrow$$
$$7,9\ 0\ 0$$

Rounding is used a great deal in health care. Rounding of whole numbers exists in inventory and packaging of supplies as well as in daily activities.

Practice   1. Round to the nearest 10:

     a. 3,918   **c.** 6,952   **e.** 15,932

     b. 139   **d.** 1,925   **f.** 99

2. Round to the nearest 100:

     a. 3,918   **c.** 8,975   **e.** 35,292

     b. 3,784   **d.** 17,854   **f.** 1,925

3. Round to the nearest 1,000:

     a. 3,190   **c.** 6,950   **e.** 432,500

     b. 87,987   **d.** 12,932   **f.** 2,987

Additional rounding practice will be presented in Unit 4: Decimals.

Estimation

Estimation is a method of coming up with a math answer that is general not specific. When we estimate, we rely on rounding to help us get to this general answer. For example, with money, rounding is done to the nearest dollar. If an amount has 50 cents or more, round to the nearest dollar and drop the cent amount. If an amount is under 50 cents, retain the dollar amount and drop the cent amount.

Example   Estimate Bob's expenses for his co-payment of his dental expenses for his two six-month checkups.

	Actual Expense	Estimated Expense
March	$65.85	$66
October	$59.10	$59

Add the estimated expenses of $66 + $59 = _____
The estimated annual total is $125.
So estimation is a skill that uses rounding to reach a general rather than a specific answer.

Practice   1. Find the sum using estimation to the nearest dollar:

     a. $56.90 + $12.45 + $124.78

     b. $127.46 + $13.98 + $21.20

     c. $23.45 + $32.29 + $56.65

     d. $2,900.87 + $12.89

2. Find the sum using estimation to the nearest hour:

    a. 1 hour 25 minutes + 2 hours 14 minutes + 5 hours 37 minutes

    b. 7 hours 8 minutes + 10 hours 34 minutes + 15 hours 45 minutes

    c. 3 hours 35 minutes + 22 hours 16 minutes + 9 hours 59 minutes

    d. 6 hours 39 minutes + 13 hours 18 minutes + 5 hours 2 minutes

Averages

Review An average is a number that represents a group of the same unit of measure. It provides a general number that represents this group of numbers if all the numbers were the same units. Averages are useful in health occupations because they provide general trends and information. Averages are computed using addition and division skills.

    To compute an average, follow these two steps:

Step 1: Add the individual units of measure.

Step 2: Divide the sum of the units of measure by the number of individual units.

Example Mary Ann wanted to know the average score of her anatomy and physiology tests. Her scores were: 92%, 79%, 100%, 89% and 95%.

Step 1: $92 + 79 + 100 + 89 + 95 = 455$

Step 2: There were a total of 5 grades.

Mary Ann's average score was 91%.

$$
\begin{array}{r}
91 \\
5\overline{)455} \\
45\downarrow \\
\hline
5 \\
5 \\
\hline
0
\end{array}
$$

Practice 1. Deb needed to purchase new calendars for the examination rooms. Find the average if the calendars cost: $11, $7, $10, $5, $10, $12, $8, and $9.

2. Certified nursing assistants work a varied number of hours every week at Village Nursing Home. The weekly hours are 32, 38, 40, 35, 40, 16, and 30. What is the average number of hours each assistant works?

3. The staff phone use during morning break is increasing. The director is considering adding additional phones and is researching the usage in minutes. Using the following data, compute the average length of each call: 7, 4, 3, 1, 2, 4, 5, 7, and 12.

4. A diabetic patient is counting calories. The patient adds up calories from portions of fruit: 90, 80, 60, 15, 40. What is the average caloric intake from each portion?

WHOLE NUMBER SELF-TEST

1. $329 + 1,075 + 217 =$

2. An activity director in a long-term care facility is purchasing recreational supplies. Find the sum of the purchases: 3 Bingo games at $13 each, 10 puzzles at $9 each, 24 jars of paint at $3 each, and 2 rolls of paper for $31 each.

3. Using the information from problem 2 above, determine the average cost of these supplies. Round to the nearest dollar.

4. A medical assistant student needs 250 hours of practical work experience to complete the college's course. If the student has completed 184 hours, how many remain to fulfill the requirement?

5. Three certified nursing assistants assist 16 rooms of patients on the Saturday morning shift. If each room has 3 patients, how many does each assistant care for if the patients are equally divided up among the staff?

6. Uniform jackets are required at Valley Pharmacy. Each pharmacy technician is asked to purchased two jackets at $21 per jacket and one name badge for $8. What is the cost of these items for each pharmacy technician?

7. The medical clerk is asked to inventory the digital thermometers. In the six examination rooms, the clerk finds the following number of digital thermometers: 2, 4, 5, 2, 1, and 3. The total inventory is _____.

8. The dental assistants in a new office are setting up their free patient sample display. The dental assistants order:

	Quantity	Unit	Item	Per Unit Cost	Total
a.	1,500	each	toothbrush	$1	_____
b.	100	each	floss-smooth	$2	_____
c.	75	each	floss-glide	$2	_____
d.	1,000	per 100	information booklet	$10	_____
e.	25	each	poster	$15	_____
f.				Subtotal	_____

9. After a mild heart attack, Mary spent 3 days in a coronary care unit. Her room bill was $2,898. What was her daily room rate?

10. White blood cell count can indicate illness or health. The white blood count (WBC) of patient B is checked. Before surgery, the white blood count (WBC) of patient B was 12,674; post-surgery, he had a count of 6,894. What is the difference in patient B's count before and after surgery?

11. The cook has a variety of meals to prepare for Villa Center's residents. She averages 16 vegetarian meals every day of the week. Round the number of weekly meals to the nearest 10.

12. The newest staff member at the hospital is a surgery technologist. Her pay is approximately $14 an hour. If she is scheduled to work 36 hours a week, what is her weekly pay before deductions?

13. Read the number: 9 5 6,123.

The place value of the underlined digit is _____.

14. Round to the nearest 10:   8,905   _____

15. Round to the nearest 100:   31,387   _____

Unit 3

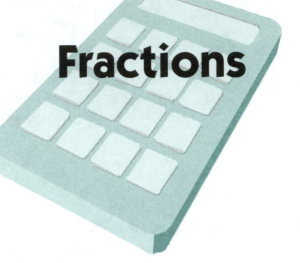

Part-to-Whole Relationships

A fraction is a number that has two parts: a part and a whole. A minute is 1 part of 60 minutes in a whole hour. This relationship of part to whole can be shown in a fraction:

$$\frac{1}{60} \quad \begin{array}{l} \leftarrow \text{numerator (the part)} \\ \leftarrow \text{denominator (the whole)} \end{array}$$

The 1 is called the numerator, and it represents the part of the whole. The 60 is the denominator, and it represents the whole or sum of the parts. Take another common part-to-whole relationship. Many people sleep an average of 8 hours a night. The relationship of sleeping hours to total hours in a day is 8 to 24, or $\frac{8}{24}$, or a reduced fraction of $\frac{1}{3}$.

Fractions are important to know because you will come across them many times in health care occupations. Fractions appear in medication dosages, measurements, sizes of instruments, work assignments, and time units. Practice writing out the numerator (part) to denominator (whole) relationships:

Example

$$\frac{1}{12} = \text{one part to twelve total parts}$$

24

1. $\dfrac{3}{4}$ = _____

2. $\dfrac{5}{6}$ = _____

3. $\dfrac{7}{8}$ = _____

4. $\dfrac{16}{21}$ = _____

Proper or common fractions are fractions with a numerator less than the number of the denominator: $^3/_7$, $^{24}/_{47}$, $^9/_{11}$. The value of any proper or common fraction will be less than 1.

Mixed numbers are fractions that include both a whole number and a proper fraction: $3\,^3/_4$, $12\,^9/_{11}$, $101\,^{13}/_{22}$.

An improper fraction has a numerator equal to or larger than the denominator: $^{17}/_{12}$, $^{33}/_{11}$, $^9/_9$. Improper fractions are equal to 1 or larger. Improper fractions will be used in the multiplication and division of fractions. Answers that appear as improper fractions will need to be reduced so that the answer is a mixed number.

Equivalent Fractions

Understanding equivalent fractions is important in making measurement decisions. Equivalent fractions represent the same relationship of part to whole, but there are more pieces or parts involved. The fractions involved, however, are equal. The size of the pieces or parts is what varies.

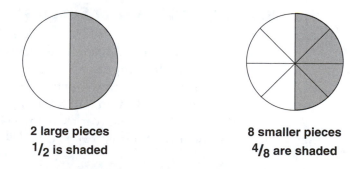

2 large pieces
$^1/_2$ is shaded

8 smaller pieces
$^4/_8$ are shaded

The shaded areas are the same size; the number of parts varies. Making fractions equal is easy using multiplication. Look at the fractions: $^1/_6$ and $^?/_{18}$. The denominators are 6 and 18. Ask: 6 times what = 18? The answer is 3, so multiply the numerator by 3, and you will have formed an equivalent fraction. Thus, $^1/_6 = ^3/_{18}$.

The key to getting the correct answer is in remembering that the number the denominator is multiplied by must also be used to multiply the numerator. If this method is difficult for you, you can also divide the smaller denominator into the larger one; your answer will then be multiplied by the first numerator to get the second numerator.

$$\frac{1}{6} = \frac{?}{18} \qquad 6\overline{)18,} \qquad \text{then} \quad 3 \times 1 = 3$$

Another way to work this problem is:

$$\frac{1 \, (\times 3)}{6 \, (\times 3)} = \frac{3}{18}$$

Thus, $\frac{1}{6} = \frac{3}{18}$.

Practice   1. $\dfrac{1}{2} = \dfrac{?}{12}$ 6. $\dfrac{1}{13} = \dfrac{?}{39}$

2. $\dfrac{1}{4} = \dfrac{?}{16}$ 7. $\dfrac{4}{8} = \dfrac{?}{72}$

3. $\dfrac{1}{5} = \dfrac{?}{40}$ 8. $\dfrac{1}{5} = \dfrac{?}{100}$

4. $\dfrac{2}{14} = \dfrac{?}{28}$ 9. $\dfrac{7}{9} = \dfrac{42}{?}$

5. $\dfrac{5}{9} = \dfrac{?}{27}$ 10. $\dfrac{1}{3} = \dfrac{8}{?}$

The skill of making equivalent fractions will be used in adding, subtracting, and comparing fractions.

Reducing to Lowest or Simplest Terms

As in making fractions equivalent, reducing fractions to their lowest or simplest terms is another important fraction skill. Most tests and practical applications of fractions require that the answers be in the lowest terms. After each calculation of addition, subtraction, multiplication, or division, you will need to reduce the answer to its lowest terms. Two methods will help you get to the lowest terms:

Multiplication Method

To use the multiplication method, look at the numbers in the fraction. Find one number that divides into both the numerator and denominator evenly. Such numbers are called factors of the numbers. Write out the multiplication for the numerator and denominator. Cross out the two identical numbers in the multiplication problems. What is left will be the reduced fraction.

$$\frac{2}{16} = \frac{2 \times 1}{2 \times 8} \rightarrow \frac{\cancel{2} \times 1}{\cancel{2} \times 8}$$

So, $^2/_{16} = {}^1/_8$. Depending on the multiple you choose, you may need to do this more than once.

$$\frac{8}{24} = \frac{\cancel{4} \times 2}{\cancel{4} \times 6} = \frac{2}{6} \rightarrow \frac{1}{3}$$

or

$$\frac{8}{24} = \frac{\cancel{8} \times 1}{\cancel{8} \times 3} = \frac{1}{3}$$

Sometimes students only partially reduce a fraction, so try to find the largest possible factor of the numbers when you are reducing.

> Choose the largest possible multiple to avoid having to repeat the steps in reduction.

Division Method

Look at the numbers of the numerator and the denominator. Choose a number that divides into both the numerator and the denominator. Next, divide the numerator and denominator by that number. Check to ensure that the resulting fraction is in its lowest form.

$$\frac{2}{16} = \frac{2 \div 2}{16 \div 2} = \frac{1}{8}$$

$$\frac{8}{24} = \frac{8 \div 4}{24 \div 4} = \frac{2}{6}$$

This fraction is not reduced, so it must be reduced again.

$$\frac{2}{6} = \frac{2 \div 2}{6 \div 2} = \frac{1}{3}$$

This fraction is reduced to its lowest form.
How do you decide on the best method to use?

> Choose your strongest skill—multiplication or division—and use it to reduce fractions.

You will make fewer errors if you select one method and use it consistently.

Practice

1. $\dfrac{2}{14}$

2. $\dfrac{3}{27}$

3. $\dfrac{4}{8}$

6. $\dfrac{64}{72}$

7. $\dfrac{24}{48}$

8. $\dfrac{63}{90}$

4. $\dfrac{13}{39}$ 9. $\dfrac{15}{45}$

5. $\dfrac{25}{100}$ 10. $\dfrac{5}{255}$

When working with a mixed number, set aside the whole number. Handle the fraction portion of the number and then place it beside the whole number.

$$14\tfrac{3}{9} \rightarrow 14 \quad \text{and} \quad \tfrac{3}{9} \rightarrow \dfrac{3}{9} = \dfrac{1 \times 3}{3 \times 3} = \dfrac{1}{3} \rightarrow 14\tfrac{1}{3}$$

> Set aside the whole number, do the reduction, then replace the whole number next to the reduced fraction.

Practice

1. $13\tfrac{2}{8}$

2. $7\tfrac{12}{16}$

3. $1\tfrac{33}{66}$

4. $2\tfrac{2}{20}$

5. $3\tfrac{3}{12}$

6. $5\tfrac{14}{64}$

7. $2\tfrac{11}{99}$

8. $10\tfrac{30}{80}$

9. $6\tfrac{45}{90}$

10. $4\tfrac{22}{30}$

Fractional parts or relationships are common in health care.

Example   In a class of 30 people, 13 students are male and 17 are female. To write the relationship of the number of males to the total number of students, we place the part (13) over the whole (30) or total number of students.

$$\dfrac{13}{30}$$

Practice   Write the fractional part that represents the relationships of the part to the whole. Then reduce all your answers to the lowest form.

1. 50 of the 125 patients see the physical therapist each week.

2. The dietitian uses 35 6-ounce glasses and 50 8-ounce glasses at breakfast. Represent in fraction form the relationship of 6-ounce glasses to 8-ounce glasses used at breakfast.

3. 30 out of 90 patients at the short-term care facility are women. What is the fractional part of women to total patients?

4. 14 female babies and 16 male babies were born on Saturday. Express the female babies to male babies as a fraction.

5. About 500 medicine cups are used daily at a long-term care facility. The nurse claims that approximately 4,000 medicine cups are used a week. What is the day to week use rate of medicine cups?

Improper Fractions

Working with improper fractions also requires reducing fractions. An improper fraction is a fraction that has a larger numerator than a denominator.

$$\frac{16}{8} = \frac{8 \times 2 = 2}{8 \times 1 = 1} \rightarrow 2$$

If the numerator and the denominator do not have a common number by which the numbers can be multiplied, simply divide the denominator into the numerator.

$$\frac{11}{8} \qquad 8\overline{)11}^{\ 1\frac{3}{8}}$$
$$\frac{8}{3}$$

The 3 is the remainder in whole numbers. Place it on top of the divisor to form a fraction.

Improper fractions will be either whole numbers or mixed numbers.

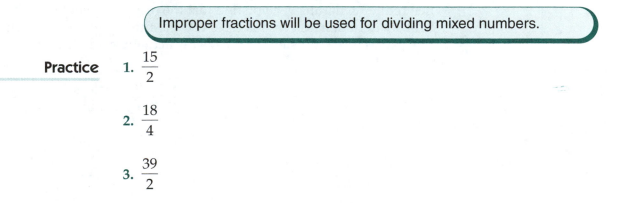

Improper fractions will be used for dividing mixed numbers.

Practice

1. $\dfrac{15}{2}$

2. $\dfrac{18}{4}$

3. $\dfrac{39}{2}$

4. $\dfrac{27}{5}$

5. $\dfrac{66}{7}$

6. $\dfrac{7}{3}$

7. $\dfrac{19}{8}$

8. $\dfrac{16}{2}$

9. $\dfrac{100}{100}$

10. $\dfrac{23}{18}$

Adding Fractions with Like Denominators

Addition of fractions with the same denominator is straightforward. Follow the two steps below:

Step 1: Line up the fractions vertically, add the numerators, and place the answer over the common, or like, denominator.

Step 2: Reduce, if necessary. Check your work to ensure accuracy.

$$\dfrac{3}{6} \qquad \dfrac{4}{8}$$
$$+\dfrac{2}{6} \qquad +\dfrac{5}{8}$$
$$\overline{5/6 \quad 9/8} \quad \text{Reduce by } 9 \div 8 = 1\tfrac{1}{8}$$

When reducing the answer, you find that the result is a whole number with a 1 for its denominator. In this case, use the numerator, a whole number alone. Do not use the 1 since the answer is actually a whole number rather than a fraction.

Step 1: $\quad \dfrac{12}{15}$
$\qquad\qquad +\dfrac{18}{15}$
$\qquad\qquad \overline{30/15}$

Step 2: $\dfrac{30}{15} = \dfrac{\cancel{15} \times 2}{\cancel{15} \times 1} \qquad \dfrac{2}{1} = 2$

If a whole number exists with the fractions, simply add it separately and place the fraction next to the answer. The whole number will be affected only if the fraction answer is larger than 1—then the whole number resulting from the fraction addition is added to the whole number answer.

Example

$$14\frac{2}{8}$$
$$+7\frac{1}{8}$$
$$\overline{21\frac{3}{8}}$$

Add the fractions: $\frac{2}{8} + \frac{1}{8} = \frac{3}{8}$

Add the whole numbers: $14 + 7 = 21$

Write the answer. No reduction is necessary.

Example

$$10\frac{2}{4}$$
$$+4\frac{3}{4}$$
$$\overline{14\frac{5}{4}}$$

Add the fractions: $\frac{2}{4} + \frac{3}{4} = \frac{5}{4}$

Add $10 + 4 = 14$

$\frac{5}{4}$ must be reduced. It is an improper fraction.

Divide 5 by $4 = 1\frac{1}{4}$. The 1, a whole number, is added to the 14 $(14 + 1 = 15)$ and the $\frac{1}{4}$ is placed next to the whole so that the answer is $15\frac{1}{4}$.

Practice   Add the following fractions. Reduce as necessary:

1. $\frac{1}{6} + \frac{5}{6}$

2. $\frac{2}{8} + \frac{4}{8}$

3. $\frac{9}{10} + \frac{11}{10}$

4. $\frac{1}{13} + \frac{4}{13}$

5. $\frac{3}{12} + \frac{4}{12}$

6. $\frac{2}{5} + \frac{3}{5}$

7. $\frac{3}{13} + \frac{4}{13}$

8. $13\frac{8}{12} + 2\frac{2}{12}$

9. $10\frac{1}{6} + 12\frac{4}{6}$

10. $11\frac{1}{4} + \frac{3}{4}$

11. $\frac{3}{5} + \frac{1}{5}$

12. $\frac{2}{7} + \frac{3}{7} + \frac{4}{7}$

13. $\frac{3}{8} + \frac{4}{8} + \frac{1}{8}$

14. $2\frac{1}{12} + 3\frac{5}{12} + 6\frac{4}{12}$

15. $101\frac{3}{4} + 33\frac{1}{4} + 5\frac{1}{4}$

Finding the Common Denominator

Adding and subtracting fractions requires that the denominator be of the same number, also referred to as a common denominator. The lowest common denominator is the smallest number or multiple that both of the denominators of the fractions can go into.

By using multiplication, find a smallest number or multiple that the numbers can go into.

Step 1:
$$\frac{2}{3} \quad \frac{}{3 \times 2 = 6} = \frac{?}{6}$$
$$+\frac{1}{6} \rightarrow \qquad \frac{1}{6}$$

In the above problem, 3 and 6 are the denominators. $3 \times 2 = 6$, so 6 is the common denominator.

Step 2: Once you have the common denominator in place, multiply the numerator by the same number with which you multiplied the denominator. The result will be equivalent fractions, so the number relationships remain the same.

$$\frac{2}{3} \quad \frac{2 \times 2 = 4}{3 \times 2 = 6}$$
$$+\frac{1}{6} \rightarrow \qquad +\frac{1}{6}$$
$$\overline{\qquad} \qquad \overline{5/6}$$

Practice Find the common denominator in the following pairs of numbers. Set the problems up vertically and think about their multiples to find the common denominators.

> Fewer errors occur if the setup is vertical. You can see the numbers and their relationships easier.

1. $\frac{2}{4}$ and $\frac{1}{5}$

2. $\frac{3}{8}$ and $\frac{1}{16}$

3. $\dfrac{22}{44}$ and $\dfrac{1}{11}$

4. $\dfrac{1}{9}$ and $\dfrac{5}{45}$

5. $\dfrac{2}{5}$ and $\dfrac{3}{25}$

6. $\dfrac{3}{7}$ and $\dfrac{9}{49}$

7. $\dfrac{1}{200}$ and $\dfrac{5}{20}$

8. $\dfrac{4}{50}$ and $\dfrac{10}{150}$

9. $\dfrac{3}{9}$ and $\dfrac{4}{27}$

10. $\dfrac{1}{6}$ and $\dfrac{4}{18}$

Practice Add the following fractions with unlike denominators:

1. $\dfrac{3}{5} + \dfrac{1}{4}$

2. $\dfrac{1}{2} + \dfrac{4}{6}$

3. $\dfrac{4}{9} + \dfrac{2}{3}$

4. $\dfrac{7}{10} + \dfrac{3}{5}$

5. $\dfrac{11}{30} + \dfrac{2}{15}$

6. $\dfrac{5}{25} + \dfrac{1}{5}$

7. $\dfrac{4}{7} + \dfrac{1}{21}$

8. $\dfrac{2}{5} + \dfrac{1}{10} + \dfrac{3}{10}$

9. $\dfrac{3}{5} + \dfrac{1}{3} + \dfrac{2}{15}$

10. $\dfrac{2}{3} + \dfrac{1}{12} + \dfrac{2}{4}$

11. $\dfrac{1}{10} + \dfrac{1}{2} + \dfrac{4}{5}$

12. $12\frac{1}{6} + \frac{3}{4}$

13. $55\frac{1}{3} + 51\frac{5}{9}$

14. $5\frac{1}{2} + 2\frac{4}{5} + 5\frac{3}{10}$

15. $4\frac{3}{4} + 1\frac{1}{16} + 3\frac{2}{32}$

Sometimes one must consider a wider range of possible numbers for common denominators. For example, you may have a pair of fractions in which one of the denominators cannot be multiplied by a number to get the other denominator. In this case, it is often easiest to simply multiply the two denominators together. The result will be a common denominator.

Example

$$\dfrac{3}{13} \quad \text{and} \quad \dfrac{1}{4}$$

What is the common denominator? If you multiply 13×4, your answer is 52. Use that number for your common denominator.

> To find the more difficult common denominators, multiply the denominators together.

$$\dfrac{3}{13} \rightarrow 13 \times 4 = 52$$

$$\dfrac{1}{4} \rightarrow 4 \times 13 = 52$$

Then multiply the numerators by the exact same number that you multiplied the denominator by. Do this for each fraction and the result will be a common denominator.

$$\dfrac{3}{13} \rightarrow \dfrac{3 \times 4 = 12}{13 \times 4 = 52}$$

$$\dfrac{1}{4} \rightarrow \dfrac{1 \times 13 = 13}{4 \times 13 = 52}$$

By making the common denominator, you have also created equivalent fractions.

Practice   Find the common denominator for each of the following sets of fractions:

1. $\dfrac{3}{4}$ and $\dfrac{2}{5}$

2. $\dfrac{7}{8}$ and $\dfrac{1}{3}$

3. $\dfrac{24}{32}$ and $\dfrac{1}{6}$

4. $\dfrac{1}{7}$ and $\dfrac{4}{8}$

5. $\dfrac{3}{5}$ and $\dfrac{7}{9}$

6. $\dfrac{2}{26}$ and $\dfrac{1}{3}$

7. $\dfrac{3}{9}$ and $\dfrac{1}{4}$

8. $\dfrac{2}{5}$ and $\dfrac{6}{9}$

9. $\dfrac{3}{10}$ and $\dfrac{2}{3}$

10. $\dfrac{1}{9}$ and $\dfrac{7}{8}$

Practice   1. $3\frac{2}{3} + 6\frac{1}{4}$

2. $10\frac{1}{2} + 13\frac{5}{22}$

3. $9\frac{1}{6} + 4\frac{3}{9}$

4. $11\frac{7}{8} + 2\frac{1}{7}$

5. $\frac{1}{2} + 4\frac{1}{7} + 2\frac{1}{14}$

6. $12\frac{3}{5} + 22\frac{1}{30}$

7. $10\frac{4}{5} + 8\frac{1}{6}$

8. $3\frac{4}{9} + 1\frac{2}{3} + 5\frac{2}{9}$

9. $11\frac{2}{5} + 7\frac{1}{2}$

10. $7\frac{11}{16} + 3\frac{4}{8} + \frac{1}{2}$

11. $2\frac{2}{9} + 6\frac{1}{3} + 8\frac{2}{27}$

12. $6\frac{2}{3} + 8\frac{4}{5} + 3\frac{6}{10}$

13. $6\frac{1}{4} + 13\frac{2}{3} + 19\frac{1}{2}$

14. $6\frac{7}{16} + \frac{3}{24} + 2\frac{1}{48}$

15. $\frac{3}{5} + \frac{6}{30} + 12\frac{2}{3}$

16. $8\frac{9}{11} + 3\frac{1}{33} + \frac{2}{66}$

17. $3\frac{5}{16} + \frac{5}{8} + \frac{2}{4}$

18. $\frac{5}{6} + 3\frac{3}{9} + 7\frac{2}{3}$

19. $4\frac{5}{6} + \frac{2}{5} + \frac{4}{15}$

20. $55\frac{4}{17} + 101\frac{3}{51}$

Applications

1. The certified nurse assistants weigh patients each month. Mrs. Smith weighed 120 pounds last month. Over the last two months, she gained $1\frac{1}{2}$ and $\frac{1}{4}$ pounds. What is Mrs. Smith's current weight?

2. The lab technician uses a cleaning solution daily. The technician used $4\frac{1}{2}$ ounces, $1\frac{1}{3}$ ounces, and 5 ounces of the cleaning solutions. What is the total amount of solution used?

3. A new baby grew $\frac{3}{4}$ of an inch in June and $\frac{7}{16}$ of an inch in July. How many total inches did the baby grow during these two months?

4. A sick child drinks $\frac{1}{2}$ cup of juice and an hour later another $\frac{3}{4}$ cup of water. At dinner, the child drinks $1\frac{1}{4}$ cups more. What is the child's total fluid intake?

5. The nurse gives a patient $1\frac{1}{2}$ grains of medication followed by $2\frac{1}{3}$ grains. What is the total dosage the nurse has dispensed to the patient?

Ordering Fractions

Comparing fractions in health care fields appears when sizes of medical items or pieces of equipment are being computed. It is useful to be able to determine the size relationships of instruments and place them in order for a surgeon prior to a surgery. This is accomplished by using the common denominator method.

Know these symbols: <, =, >

3 is less than 4 is represented by $3 < 4$

7 is greater than 5 is represented by $7 > 5$

$\frac{2}{2}$ equals 1 is represented by $\frac{2}{2} = 1$

Example Which is larger $\frac{1}{4}$ or $\frac{3}{8}$?

Step 1: Convert the fractions to give each a common denominator.

$$\frac{1}{4} \qquad \frac{1 \times 2 = 2}{4 \times 2 = 8}$$

$$\frac{3}{8} \rightarrow \qquad \frac{3}{8}$$

Step 2: Order by the numerators now that the fractions have the same denominator. 3 is larger than 2, so $\frac{3}{8} > \frac{2}{8}$ or $\frac{1}{4}$.

Practice Order the following fractions from largest to smallest.

1. $\dfrac{1}{4}, \dfrac{2}{9}, \dfrac{4}{12}$

2. $\dfrac{9}{22}, \dfrac{5}{11}, \dfrac{8}{11}$

3. $\dfrac{6}{25}, \dfrac{20}{50}, \dfrac{33}{100}$

4. $\dfrac{7}{8}, \dfrac{2}{16}, \dfrac{3}{4}, \dfrac{1}{2}$

Subtraction of Fractions

Subtraction of fractions follows the same basic principles as addition of fractions. The fractions must have common denominators before any subtraction can be done.

Example **Step 1:** Make a common denominator if necessary.

$$\frac{7}{8} - \frac{5}{8} = \underline{\quad} \qquad \text{(8 is the common denominator).}$$

Step 2: Subtract the numerators and then reduce if necessary.

$$\frac{7}{8} - \frac{5}{8} = \frac{2}{8}, \text{ which is reduced to } \frac{1}{4}.$$

Practice   1. $\dfrac{3}{9} - \dfrac{2}{9}$

2. $\dfrac{5}{8} - \dfrac{2}{8}$

3. $\dfrac{3}{11} - \dfrac{1}{11}$

4. $\dfrac{22}{44} - \dfrac{11}{44}$

5. $10^5\!/_{12} - 8^3\!/_{12}$

6. $25^3\!/_4 - 20^1\!/_4$

7. $101^{13}\!/_{24} - 56^{10}\!/_{24}$

8. $6^6\!/_7 - ^3\!/_5$

9. $\dfrac{15}{16} - \dfrac{7}{16}$

10. $20^5\!/_6 - 12^2\!/_6$

11. $\dfrac{3}{4} - \dfrac{1}{2}$

12. $\dfrac{6}{8} - \dfrac{1}{4}$

13. $12^1\!/_2 - ^3\!/_{10}$

14. $20^6\!/_{14} - 2^3\!/_7$

15. $39^{11}\!/_{18} - 8^3\!/_6$

16. $25^1\!/_3 - 20^1\!/_8$

17. $124^{11}\!/_{12} - ^5\!/_6$

18. $18^3\!/_4 - 12^2\!/_3$

19. $200^9\!/_{11} - 188^2\!/_3$

20. $500^4\!/_5 - 150^2\!/_9$

Borrowing in Subtraction of Fractions

Two specific situations require that a number be borrowed in the subtraction of fractions: (1) subtraction of a fraction from a whole number, and (2) after a common denominator is established and the top fraction of the problem is less or smaller than the fraction that is being subtracted from it.

Recall that the borrowing in whole numbers is accomplished as shown below. Set the problem up vertically.

$$124 - 8 = \underline{\hspace{1cm}}$$

Step 1: Borrow 1 from the tens column. Add it to the ones column.

Step 2: Subtract.

$$
\begin{array}{r}
1^{1}\!\!\not2^{1}4 \\
-\ 8 \\
\hline
116
\end{array}
$$

In fractions, the same borrowing concept is used; the format varies only slightly. The difference is that the borrowed number must be put into a fractional form.

> Any whole number over itself equals 1. So $^{101}\!/_{101} = 1$, $^{3}\!/_{3} = 1$, and $^{12}\!/_{12} = 1$.

Example

$$
\begin{array}{r}
17\dfrac{3}{8} \\[2ex]
-14\dfrac{4}{8} \\
\hline
\end{array}
$$

In the example above, the 4 in the second fraction's numerator cannot be subtracted from the 3. Thus, borrowing is required.

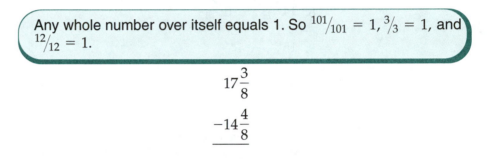

$$
\begin{array}{r}
1^{6}\!\!\not7\dfrac{3}{8} + \dfrac{8}{8} \\[2ex]
-14\dfrac{4}{8} \\
\hline
\end{array}
$$

Step 1: Borrow 1 from the whole number. Convert the 1 into a fraction. Use the same number as the common denominator. Put the common denominator over itself, then add it to the existing denominator.

Step 2: Rewrite the problem so it incorporates the changes, then subtract the numerator only. Place it over the denominator. Reduce as necessary.

$$
\begin{array}{r}
16\dfrac{11}{8} \\[2ex]
14\dfrac{4}{8} \\
\hline
2^{7}\!/_{8}
\end{array}
$$

> ### Borrowing in Subtraction Rules
> 1. Must have a common denominator.
> 2. To borrow from the whole number, make it a fractional part.
> 3. Add fractional parts.
> 4. Subtract; reduce if necessary.

Practice

1. $11 - \frac{5}{6}$

2. $9 - \frac{3}{5}$

3. $10 - \frac{2}{8}$

4. $13 - \frac{5}{9}$

5. $15 - \frac{7}{13}$

6. $30 - \frac{4}{11}$

7. $8\frac{2}{7} - 2\frac{3}{7}$

8. $14\frac{3}{12} - 10\frac{10}{12}$

9. $15\frac{1}{5} - 4\frac{4}{5}$

10. $9\frac{2}{4} - 5\frac{3}{4}$

Remember that when you are subtracting, the first rule is that you must have a common denominator. Once the common denominator is in place, borrow if necessary. Then subtract, placing the answer over the denominator; reduce as necessary.

Practice

1. $14\frac{2}{5} - 6\frac{3}{4}$

2. $34\frac{1}{4} - 10\frac{4}{5}$

3. $36\frac{1}{6} - 16\frac{3}{5}$

4. $13\frac{3}{4} - 7\frac{7}{8}$

5. $16\frac{3}{11} - 10\frac{1}{2}$

6. $19\frac{1}{2} - 15\frac{7}{12}$

7. $112\frac{1}{2} - \frac{11}{15}$

8. $18\frac{3}{7} - 2\frac{7}{14}$

9. $45\frac{3}{8} - 13\frac{3}{4}$

10. $125\frac{2}{12} - 28\frac{5}{6}$

11. $29\frac{1}{4} - 12\frac{5}{12}$

12. $12\frac{1}{6} - 1\frac{4}{5}$

13. $90\frac{4}{9} - 13\frac{3}{4}$

14. $28\frac{1}{7} - 4\frac{6}{7}$

15. $13\frac{2}{20} - 6\frac{6}{10}$

Application

1. A patient is on a low sodium, low fat diet. Three months ago the patient weighed $210\frac{1}{4}$ pounds. Now the patient weighs $198\frac{3}{4}$ pounds. How many pounds did the patient lose?

2. The school nurse encourages all students to drink at least 4 pints of water daily. Most students drink at least $1\frac{1}{2}$ pints. How much additional water should the students consume?

3. The pharmacy technician helps with annual inventory. If there were 125 boxes of computer labels at the beginning of the inventory period, and $25\frac{3}{4}$ remain, how many boxes of labels were used throughout the year?

4. The dietitian had a 100 pound bag of unbleached flour at the beginning of the month. If she used $73\frac{1}{2}$ pounds, how much flour does she have left?

5. The recreation center is helping residents make placemats for the holidays. Each resident is given 45 inches of decorative edging per placemat. If each placemat uses $41\frac{1}{2}$ inches of decorative edging, how much edging is left over from each placemat?

Multiplication of Fractions

To facilitate multiplication and division of fractions, set up the problems horizontally.

One of the simplest computations in fractions is to multiply a common fraction. No common denominator is needed.

Example

Step 1: Set up the problem horizontally and multiply the fraction straight across.

$$\frac{7 \times 1 \rightarrow}{8 \times 4 \rightarrow} = \frac{7}{32}$$

Step 2: Reduce to the lowest terms, if necessary. $\frac{7}{32}$ does not need to be reduced.

Practice

1. $\frac{3}{4} \times \frac{1}{12}$

2. $\frac{1}{2} \times \frac{4}{5}$

3. $\dfrac{7}{9} \times \dfrac{4}{5}$

4. $\dfrac{2}{3} \times \dfrac{4}{6}$

5. $\dfrac{1}{5} \times \dfrac{3}{7}$

6. $\dfrac{12}{48} \times \dfrac{1}{2}$

7. $\dfrac{6}{9} \times \dfrac{2}{3}$

8. $\dfrac{10}{100} \times \dfrac{2}{5}$

9. $\dfrac{1}{3} \times \dfrac{13}{22}$

10. $\dfrac{4}{5} \times \dfrac{1}{20}$

Review some number concepts in fractions that will help ensure accurate answers.

> Any number over itself equals 1: $^4/_4$, $^8/_8$, and $^{105}/_{105}$ all equal 1.
>
> Any numerator that has 1 as its denominator should be represented as a whole number:
>
> $$^4/_1 = 4, \, ^6/_1 = 6, \, ^{51}/_1 = 51, \text{ and } ^{102}/_1 = 102$$

Multiplying a Fraction by a Whole Number

To multiply a fraction by a whole number, follow these steps:

Example

$$\dfrac{1}{6} \times 2 = \underline{\hspace{1cm}}$$

Step 1: Make the whole number into a fraction by placing a 1 as its denominator.

$$\dfrac{1}{6} \times \dfrac{2}{1}$$

> Any whole number can become a fraction by placing a 1 as the denominator. $14 = {}^{14}/_1$

Step 2: Multiply straight across and then reduce if necessary.

$$\frac{1}{6} \times \frac{2}{1} = \frac{2}{6} \rightarrow \frac{1}{3}$$

Reduce to $\frac{1}{3}$.

Practice

1. $\frac{1}{4} \times 6$

2. $3 \times \frac{2}{5}$

3. $\frac{7}{15} \times 35$

4. $24 \times \frac{2}{7}$

5. $7 \times \frac{8}{10}$

6. $16 \times \frac{1}{3}$

7. $\frac{5}{9} \times 21$

8. $\frac{5}{30} \times 200$

9. $\frac{1}{8} \times 32$

10. $\frac{11}{50} \times 20$

Reducing before You Multiply as a Timesaver

When multiplying, you can expedite the work by reducing before you multiply. This is useful because it relies on the multiples of the numbers to reduce the numbers you are multiplying. This saves time at the end of the problem because you won't have to spend so much time reducing the answer.

Look at the numbers involved in $\frac{2}{5} \times \frac{3}{4}$. If a numerator number can go into a denominator number evenly, then canceling is possible.

$$\frac{\overset{1}{\cancel{2}}}{5} \times \frac{3}{\underset{2}{\cancel{4}}} \qquad \text{The 2 goes into the 4 twice because } 2 \times 2 = 4.$$

Then multiply the changed numerals straight across.

$$\frac{1 \times 3 =}{5 \times 2 =} \frac{3}{10}$$

The answer is $\frac{3}{10}$. If the problem was done without canceling, the answer after multiplication would be $\frac{6}{20}$, which needs to be reduced to $\frac{3}{10}$. Reducing first saves time by allowing you to work with smaller numbers. For more complicated problems, it may be easier to cancel by writing out the number involved.

Example   **Step 1:** Write out the multiples of each number to find numbers that each can go into evenly.

$$(10 \times 1) \qquad (3 \times 1)$$
$$\frac{10}{15} \quad \times \quad \frac{3}{100}$$
$$(3 \times 5) \qquad (10 \times 10)$$

Step 2: Then, begin by crossing out the matching numbers, working from top to bottom and crossing out like numbers. Cross out the matching numbers.

$$(\cancel{10} \times 1) \qquad (\cancel{3} \times 1)$$
$$\frac{10}{15} \quad \times \quad \frac{3}{100}$$
$$(\cancel{3} \times 5) \qquad (\cancel{10} \times 10)$$

Step 3: Then multiply the remaining numbers straight across.

$$(\cancel{10} \times 1) \qquad (\cancel{3} \times 1) \qquad \rightarrow 1 \times 1 = \underline{1}$$
$$\frac{10}{15} \quad \times \quad \frac{3}{100} \qquad\qquad\qquad\qquad \left.\right\}\frac{1}{50}$$
$$(\cancel{3} \times 5) \qquad (\cancel{10} \times 10) \qquad \rightarrow 5 \times 10 = 50$$

Practice

1. $\dfrac{4}{5} \times \dfrac{15}{7}$

2. $\dfrac{12}{20} \times \dfrac{4}{24}$

3. $\dfrac{3}{7} \times \dfrac{21}{36}$

4. $\dfrac{5}{6} \times \dfrac{3}{30}$

5. $\dfrac{11}{15} \times \dfrac{3}{44}$

6. $\dfrac{3}{7} \times \dfrac{7}{11}$

7. $\dfrac{14}{20} \times \dfrac{10}{28}$

8. $\dfrac{1}{3} \times \dfrac{3}{6} \times \dfrac{2}{4}$

9. $\dfrac{11}{16} \times \dfrac{4}{12} \times \dfrac{22}{44}$

10. $\dfrac{9}{10} \times \dfrac{1}{3} \times \dfrac{8}{13}$

Multiplication of Mixed Numbers

Mixed numbers are whole numbers with fractions. Multiplication involving mixed numbers requires that the mixed number be changed to an improper fraction.

Example Change $1\frac{3}{4}$ into an improper fraction.

Step 1: Multiply the whole number times the denominator, then add the numerator.

$$1 \times 4 = 4 + 3 = 7$$

Step 2: Place the answer from step 1 over the denominator.

$$\frac{7}{4} \qquad \text{So } 1\frac{3}{4} = \frac{7}{4}$$

These improper fractions are not further reduced or changed. They may now be multiplied by another fraction.

Practice Change these mixed numbers into improper fractions.

1. $8\frac{1}{4}$

2. $5\frac{2}{3}$

3. $17\frac{3}{5}$

4. $24\frac{4}{7}$

5. $2\frac{3}{12}$

6. $4\frac{3}{8}$

7. $3\frac{5}{9}$

8. $12\frac{1}{4}$

9. $4\frac{5}{12}$

10. $10\frac{1}{3}$

After converting mixed numbers to improper fractions, continue by following the same rules as for multiplying common fractions.

Example

$$\frac{1}{3} \times 5\frac{1}{4}$$

Step 1: Change the mixed number into improper fractions.

$$5\frac{1}{4} \rightarrow 5 \times 4 = 20 + 1 = \frac{21}{4}$$

Step 2: Cancel, if possible.

$$\frac{1}{3} \quad \times \quad \frac{\overset{(3 \times 7)}{21}}{4}$$
$$(3 \times 1)$$

Step 3: Multiply straight across.

$$\frac{1 \times 7 = 7}{1 \times 4 = 4}$$

Step 4: Reduce as necessary.

$$\frac{7}{4} \rightarrow 7 \div 4 = 1\frac{3}{4}$$

Example

$$3\frac{1}{4} \times 5\frac{2}{5}$$

Step 1: Change to improper fractions.

$$3\frac{1}{4} \rightarrow 3 \times 4 = 12 + 1 = \frac{13}{4} \quad \text{and}$$

$$5\frac{2}{5} \rightarrow 5 \times 5 = 25 + 2 = \frac{27}{5}$$

Step 2: Cancel, if possible.

$$\frac{13}{4} \times \frac{27}{5} \text{—not possible}$$

Step 3: Multiply straight across.

$$\frac{13 \times 27}{4 \times 5} = \frac{351}{20}$$

Step 4: Reduce → Divide 351 by 20.

$$\begin{array}{r} 17\,^{11}/_{20} \\ 20\overline{)351} \\ \underline{20\downarrow} \\ 151 \\ \underline{140} \\ 11 \end{array}$$
      Answer: $17\,^{11}/_{20}$

Practice

1. $2\,^{5}/_{12} \times \,^{1}/_{7}$

2. $4\,^{2}/_{3} \times \,^{4}/_{5}$

3. $^{3}/_{10} \times 1\,^{3}/_{4}$

4. $2\,^{1}/_{8} \times \,^{6}/_{11}$

5. $^{4}/_{9} \times 1\,^{2}/_{3}$

6. $3\,^{5}/_{7} \times 2\,^{5}/_{14}$

7. $17\,^{1}/_{4} \times 2\,^{1}/_{3}$

8. $1\,^{1}/_{4} \times 2\,^{1}/_{5}$

9. $2\,^{1}/_{5} \times 1\,^{3}/_{4}$

10. $3\,^{1}/_{6} \times 3\,^{1}/_{4}$

Applications

1. A bottle of medicine contains 30 doses. How many doses are in $2\,^{1}/_{3}$ bottles?

2. The nurse worked a total of $2\,^{1}/_{4}$ hours overtime. She is paid \$32 an hour for overtime work. What are her overtime earnings?

3. One tablet contains 250 milligrams of pain medication. How many milligrams are in $3\frac{1}{2}$ tablets?

4. One cup holds 8 ounces of liquid. If a cup is $\frac{2}{3}$ full, how many ounces are in the cup?

5. The dietitian is working in a long-term care residence. Each day she prepares a high protein drink for 25 residents. If each drink measures $\frac{3}{4}$ cup, how many total cups of the drink will she prepare a day?

Division of Fractions

To divide fractions, two steps are required to compute the answer.

Example   **Step 1:** Invert the fraction to the right of the ÷ sign.

$$\frac{1}{8} \div \frac{1}{4} \rightarrow \frac{1}{8} \div \frac{4}{1}$$

This inversion causes the fraction to change from $\frac{1}{4}$ to $\frac{4}{1}$, which is called the reciprocal of $\frac{1}{4}$.

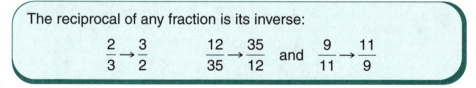

The reciprocal of any fraction is its inverse:

$$\frac{2}{3} \rightarrow \frac{3}{2} \qquad \frac{12}{35} \rightarrow \frac{35}{12} \quad \text{and} \quad \frac{9}{11} \rightarrow \frac{11}{9}$$

Step 2: Once the inversion is complete, change the sign to a × sign.

$$\frac{1}{8} \div \frac{1}{4} \rightarrow \frac{1}{8} \div \frac{4}{1} \rightarrow \frac{1}{8} \times \frac{4}{1}$$

Step 3: Follow the steps of multiplication of fractions: Cancel if possible; multiply straight across and reduce as necessary.

$$\frac{1}{8} \times \frac{4}{1} = \frac{4}{8} \qquad \text{Reduce to } \frac{1}{2}$$

$$\frac{4}{9} \div \frac{1}{3} =$$

Example   **Step 1:** Invert the fraction after the ÷ sign.

$$\frac{4}{9} \div \frac{3}{1}$$

Step 2: Change the ÷ sign to an × sign.

$$\frac{4}{9} \times \frac{3}{1}$$

Step 3: Multiply straight across.

Reduce

$$\frac{4}{9} \times \frac{3}{1} = \frac{12}{9} \qquad \begin{array}{r} 1\,^3\!/_9 \\ 9\overline{)12} \\ \underline{-9} \end{array}$$

The answer is $1\,^3\!/_9$. Note $^3\!/_9$ reduces to $^1\!/_3$, so the answer is $1\,^1\!/_3$.

> Whole numbers require placing a 1 as a denominator prior to any division or multiplication of their digits.

Practice   **1.** $\dfrac{3}{7} \div \dfrac{3}{5}$

2. $\dfrac{5}{35} \div \dfrac{11}{21}$

3. $\dfrac{3}{12} \div \dfrac{6}{7}$

4. $\dfrac{7}{9} \div \dfrac{4}{5}$

5. $\dfrac{8}{9} \div \dfrac{1}{9}$

6. $33 \div \dfrac{11}{12}$

7. $\dfrac{1}{3} \div 15$

8. $6 \div \dfrac{1}{3}$

9. $\dfrac{7}{28} \div 30$

10. $8\frac{6}{10} \div 1\frac{4}{5}$

11. $4\frac{3}{8} \div 1\frac{2}{16}$

12. $7\frac{1}{2} \div 3\frac{1}{5}$

13. $12\frac{4}{8} \div 4\frac{1}{2}$

14. $12\frac{4}{10} \div 3\frac{1}{3}$

15. $5\frac{1}{2} \div 1\frac{1}{8}$

16. $3\frac{5}{8} \div 2\frac{1}{2}$

17. $2\frac{3}{14} \div 9\frac{2}{7}$

18. $1\frac{7}{9} \div \frac{8}{11}$

19. $10\frac{6}{7} \div 7\frac{1}{2}$

20. $1\frac{9}{12} \div \frac{1}{12}$

Applications

1. A lab technician worked $45\frac{3}{4}$ hours in 5 days. He worked the same number of hours each day. How many hours a day did he work?

2. How many $\frac{1}{4}$ gram doses can be obtained from a $7\frac{1}{2}$ gram vial of medication?

3. The pharmacy technician's paycheck was for $1,123.85. If the technician worked $84\frac{1}{2}$ hours, what is the hourly rate of pay?

4. The nurse must give a patient 9 milligrams of a medication. If the tablets are 2 milligrams each, how many tablets are needed?

5. The pharmacy has 5 gram vials of medication. How many $\frac{1}{2}$ gram doses are available?

Fraction Formula

Memorize these two setups:

To convert Fahrenheit to Celsius: $°F - 32 \times {}^5/_9 = °C$

To convert Celsius to Fahrenheit: $°C \times {}^9/_5 + 32 = °F$

Follow these steps to change a Fahrenheit temperature to a Celsius temperature:

Example $5°C = \underline{\hspace{1cm}} °F$

Step 1:

$$°C \times \frac{9}{5} \rightarrow \quad 5 \times \frac{9}{5} = \frac{45}{5} \qquad 5\overline{)45} = 9 \;\; \frac{9}{}$$
$$\underline{45}$$

Step 2: Add 32 to the step 1 answer to get the °C.

$$9 + 32 = 41 \;°F$$

> Fractions are used to convert between Celsius and Fahrenheit temperatures. Fractions are more accurate than decimals because there is no change in the numbers as a result of the rounding of decimals.

Practice   **1.** $20°C = \underline{\hspace{1cm}} °F$

2. $35°C = \underline{\hspace{1cm}} °F$

3. $25°C = \underline{\hspace{1cm}} °F$

4. $60°C = \underline{\hspace{1cm}} °F$

5. $40°C = \underline{\hspace{1cm}} °F$

6. $45°C = \underline{\hspace{1cm}} °F$

7. $80°C = \underline{\hspace{1cm}} °F$

8. $15°C = \underline{\hspace{1cm}} °F$

Follow these steps to change a Celsius temperature to a Fahrenheit temperature:

Example $122°F = \underline{\hspace{1cm}} °C$

Step 1: $°F - 32 = \underline{\hspace{1cm}}$ Subtract 32 from the
                   $122°F$ Fahrenheit temperature.
                   $\underline{-32}$
                   90

Step 2: Multiply step 1 answer by $^5/_9$ to get the °C.

$$90 \times \frac{5}{9} = \frac{450}{9} \qquad \text{Divide 450 by 9.}$$

$$\begin{array}{r} 50 \\ 9\overline{)450} \\ 45\downarrow \\ \hline 00 \end{array}$$

So, 122°F is 50°C.

Practice   **1.** 104°F = _____ °C

2. 32°F = _____ °C

3. 50°F = _____ °C

4. 113°F = _____ °C

5. 59°F = _____ °C

6. 131°F = _____ °C

7. 86°F = _____ °C

8. 59°F = _____ °C

Some temperatures will require working with decimals. Additional practice will be provided in Unit 4: Decimals.

Complex Fractions

Complex fractions are used to help nurses and pharmacy technicians compute exact dosages. Complex fractions may also more efficiently solve difficult problems. A complex fraction is a fraction within a fraction.

Example $\dfrac{1/4}{6} \nwarrow \quad \dfrac{3/4}{1/100} \nwarrow \quad$ These fraction lines should be viewed as a division sign.

Complex fractions are solved by using the rules of division. These examples become:

$$\frac{1}{4} \div 6 \rightarrow \frac{1}{4} \div \frac{6}{1} \rightarrow \frac{1}{4} \times \frac{1}{6} = \frac{1}{24}$$

$$\frac{3}{4} \div \frac{1}{100} \rightarrow \frac{3}{4} \div \frac{1}{100} \rightarrow \frac{3}{4} \times \frac{100}{1} = \frac{300}{4} \qquad \text{Reduce to } \frac{75}{1} = 75$$

Practice Solve these complex fractions. Reduce to the lowest terms.

1. $\dfrac{3/8}{4}$

6. $\dfrac{3/4}{2/3}$

2. $\dfrac{1/8}{100}$

7. $\dfrac{1/125}{2/200}$

3. $\dfrac{1/300}{50}$

8. $\dfrac{1/2}{1/4}$

4. $\dfrac{40}{1/25}$

9. $\dfrac{1/80}{1/75}$

5. $\dfrac{1/50}{1/60}$

10. $\dfrac{1/10}{1/100}$

Dosage problems will also combine complex fractions with whole numbers and decimal numbers to compute the correct dosage. This work will be further covered in Unit 8: Dosage Calculations.

Example

$$\dfrac{1/300}{1/100} \times 200$$

These types of problems appear more difficult than they actually are. Group the work into sections so that it is manageable, and you can track your progress.

Step 1: Handle the complex fraction first by dividing it.

$$\frac{1}{300} \div \frac{1}{100} \rightarrow \frac{1}{300} \times \frac{100}{1} = \frac{100}{300} \rightarrow \text{Reduce to } 1/3$$

Step 2: Next, rewrite the entire problem.

$$\frac{1}{3} \times 200 \qquad \text{Then work this portion of the problem.}$$

$$\frac{1}{3} \times \frac{200}{1} = \frac{200}{3} \qquad \text{Reduce by dividing 200 by 3.}$$

The answer is $66\frac{2}{3}$. If the problem has a fraction it in, the answer may have a fraction in it. Do not convert this fraction to a decimal number.

Practice   Solve these problems.

1. $\dfrac{5/8}{1/4} \times 2$

3. $\dfrac{15/500}{1/100} \times 4$

2. $\dfrac{1/200}{1/100} \times 80$

4. $\dfrac{1/125}{1/500} \times 25$

FRACTION SELF-TEST

Reduce all answers to lowest terms.

1. A day has 24 hours. 6 hours is what fractional part of the 24 hours?

2. Write two equivalent fractions for $\dfrac{1}{6}$.

3. Reduce $\dfrac{122}{11}$

4. $8\frac{1}{6} + 3\frac{3}{4}$

5. $52 - 12\frac{1}{5}$

6. $14\frac{1}{2} \times 2\frac{1}{8}$

7. $5\frac{2}{6} \div 12$

8. $77°\,\text{F} = \underline{}°\,\text{C}$

9. Order from smallest to largest: $\dfrac{3}{8}, \dfrac{1}{3}, \dfrac{1}{4}, \dfrac{2}{12}$

10. Solve: $\qquad \dfrac{1/4}{1/8} \times 25$

11. The doctor orders grain $\frac{1}{8}$ of a medicine. The nurse has grain $\frac{1}{6}$ on hand in the medicine cabinet. Will the nurse give more or less of the dose on hand? _____

12. The physical therapist asks Mr. Smith to walk 20 minutes in one hour to improve his ambulation. What fractional part of an hour is Mr. Smith to exercise? _____

13. Among the fractions $\frac{1}{3}$, $\frac{1}{5}$, $\frac{5}{8}$ which one is equivalent to $\frac{15}{24}$? _____

14. On the dietitian's beverage tray, there are 16 filled 6-ounce glasses. Four glasses contain prune juice and two glasses contain red wine. What fractional part of the glasses contains some beverage other than prune juice or red wine? Express the answer as a fraction. _____

15. Sally works in a nursery. Her job includes recording an accurate weight for each baby. One baby weighs $7\frac{1}{3}$ pounds, two babies weigh $6\frac{1}{2}$ pounds, and a fourth baby weighs $5\frac{7}{8}$ pounds. What is the current total weight of the babies? _____

Unit 4

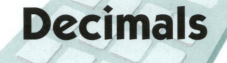

Decimals are used every day in health care settings. Understanding the application of decimals provides a strong foundation for measurement conversions, the metric system, medication dosages, and general charting work. Most medication orders are written using the metric system, which relies on decimals.

A decimal represents a part or fraction of a whole number. Decimal numbers are parts of 10s, 100s, 1000s, etc. In other words, decimals are multiples of ten. The decimal point (•) represents the boundary between whole numbers and decimal numbers.

Decimal Place Values

whole numbers					decimal numbers				
thousands	hundreds	tens	ones	and	tenths	hundredths	thousandths	ten-thousandths	hundred-thousandths
	1	0	4	•	9	9			

Consider $104.99. We understand this number to be one hundred four dollars and ninety-nine cents. The decimal point is the *and* if we write the number in words.

Any number to the left of the decimal point is always a whole number and any number to the right of the decimal point is a decimal number. Without a whole number, a decimal number is always less than 1. So we understand that 0.89 and 0.123 are less than 1.

Health care workers include a zero to the left of the decimal point for any decimal that does not include a whole number. This signals the reader that the dose, measurement, or amount is less than 1. The zero also helps avoid errors caused by misreading a decimal number. This does not change the value of the number.

Examples   0.89 and 0.123

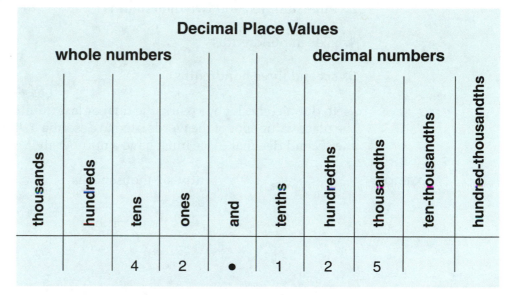

Reading decimal numbers is simple if you follow these tips: To read decimal numbers, say the numbers from left to right as if they were whole numbers, then add the decimal place value.

42.125 → read as forty-two and one hundred twenty-five thousandths.

> Identify decimal numbers by looking for the words that end in "th" or "ths."

Write the decimals in words using this method:

1. 0.7

2. 0.89

3. 0.05

4. 4.3

5. 150.075

6. 34.009

7. 125.023

8. 47.9

9. 18.08

10. 0.126

Write the following words in decimal numbers:

1. two tenths

2. thirteen thousandths

3. three hundred and two thousandths

4. sixteen hundredths

5. six and three hundredths

   To double-check your work, the final or last number should be placed in the place value spot of the words used to describe it. If it is hundredths, then the second decimal place must have a number in it.

Example

fifty-six thousandths
0.056
↑ thousandths place

Rounding Decimals

Decimals are rounded in health care to create manageable numbers. We may have a difficult time visualizing a number such as 14.39757. However, we can easily understand the number 14.4 or 14.40. Rounding to a specific decimal place is accomplished in the same way that whole numbers are rounded. In general, health care workers round decimal numbers to the nearest tenth or the nearest hundredth.

Example Round 1.75 to the nearest tenth

Step 1: Underline the place to which you are rounding

1.7̲5

Step 2: Circle one number to the right of the underlined number. If the circled number is 5 or greater, add 1 to the underlined number, and drop all the numbers to the right of the changed number. If the circled number is less than 5, do not change the underlined number, and drop all the numbers to the right of that number.

$$1.7\underline{5}\!\!⑤ \qquad \rightarrow 1.8$$

Sometimes a health care worker will round to the tenths place value, and the whole number will be affected.

Example   Round 4.97 to the nearest tenth.

Step 1:   4.<u>9</u>7

Step 2:   4.9⑦   4.9(+1) = 5.0 or 5

Practice   Round to the nearest tenth:

1. 6.74	**6.** 704.95
2. 249.86	**7.** 0.0943
3. 0.78	**8.** 349.37
4. 3.612	**9.** 9.89
5. 25.02	**10.** 0.087

Round to the nearest hundredth:

1. 17.327	**6.** $2,104.399
2. 0.975	**7.** 32.651
3. 4.8166	**8.** 9.27194
4. 0.0650	**9.** 46.085
5. 0.0074	**10.** 4.719

When and which place value to round to is a frequently asked question. General guidelines for rounding will be provided in Unit 8: Dosage Calculations.

Comparing Decimals

Comparing decimals is valuable in health occupations because many different pieces of equipment are used that may be in metric measurements. Decimals are part of the metric system, thus understanding them is necessary to determine which instrument or measurement is larger or smaller.

Comparing decimals is a skill that is also useful in sorting and ordering inventory items by size.

To compare decimals, you will rely on your eyes rather than any specific math computation.

Example Which is larger: 0.081 or 0.28?

Step 1: Line the decimals up like buttons on a shirt. This will help make the decimal numbers appear to have the same number of decimal places.

$$0.081$$
$$0.28$$

Step 2: Add zeros to fill in the empty place values so that the numbers have the same number of places or digits.

$$0.081$$
$$0.280$$

Step 3: Disregard the decimal point for a moment and read the numbers as they are written from left to right, including the added zero place values.

$$0.081 \rightarrow \text{eighty-one}$$
$$0.280 \rightarrow \text{two hundred eighty}$$

So, 0.28 is larger than 0.081.

Practice Which decimal number is smaller?

1. 0.9 or 0.89

2. 0.025 or 0.5

3. 2.12 or 2.012

4. 0.4 or 0.04

5. 0.0033 or 0.03

Which is larger?

1. 0.0785 or 0.0195

2. 0.345 or 0.35

3. 0.5 or 0.055

4. 100.75 or 100.07

5. 0.0679 or 0.675

Using the same method, arrange the sets of numbers from largest to smallest:

1. 0.75, 7.5, 0.7, 7.075, 0.07

2. 0.01, 1.01, 10.010, 1.001

3. 0.5, 5.15, 5.55, 5.05, 0.05

4. 0.04, 0.0040, 0.4, 0.044

Addition of Decimals

To add decimals, first line up the decimal points, then add. This might mean that the problem presented in a horizontal pattern may need to be rewritten in a vertical pattern.

> A whole number always has a decimal to the right side of the final number: 56 = 56.

$$2.32 + 0.14 = ? \rightarrow \begin{array}{r} 2.32 \\ + 0.14 \\ \hline 2.46 \end{array}$$

$$48 + 1.75 = \underline{} \rightarrow \begin{array}{r} 48 \\ + 1.75 \\ \hline 49.75 \end{array}$$

Lining up the decimals is the first step in ensuring the correct answer for the addition of decimals.

$$2.4\,6 + 0.005 + 1.3 = \underline{} \rightarrow \begin{array}{r} 2.46 \\ 0.005 \\ + 1.3 \\ \hline 3.765 \end{array}$$

Step 1: Line up the decimals. The order of the numbers to be added is unimportant.

Step 2: Add the numbers and bring the decimal point straight down.

Practice

1. 0.9 + 36 + 1.25

2. 15.2 + 17.071 + 0.74

3. 0.11 + 86 + 0.125

4. 10.79 + 0.99 + 0.25

5. 0.0096 + 50.24 + 39

6. 0.849 + 1.6 + 56.3

7. 14.28 + 16.24 + 97

8. 0.75 + 23.87 + 124.07

9. 13.75 + 0.001 + 200.53

10. 35.01 + 76.02 + 0.0998

Applications

1. A 25-year-old patient receives the following medication dosages daily: 1.50 milligrams, 2.25 milligrams, and 0.75 milligrams. What is his total dosage?

2. A child weighs 15.9 kilograms. The child has gained 0.9 and 1.5 kilograms during the past two months. What is the child's current weight?

3. Patient Smith receives 4 tablets of medication dosages daily: One tablet is 225 milligrams, two tablets are 0.125 milligrams each, and 1 tablet is 0.75 milligrams. What is the patient's total daily dosage of medication in milligrams?

4. One tablet is labeled 124 milligrams and another is 0.5 milligrams. What is the total dosage of these two tablets?

5. A child measured 122 centimeters in a semiannual check-up with the doctor. What would be the child's height at the next office visit if the child grew 2.54 centimeters?

Subtraction of Decimals

To subtract decimals, two steps are followed:

$$95.5 - 0.76 = \underline{\hspace{1cm}}$$

Step 1: Set the problem up vertically. Put the larger number or the number from which the second number is being subtracted on top, then line up the decimals.

$$\begin{array}{r} 95.50 \leftarrow \text{Fill in the empty places with 0s} \\ -0.76 \end{array}$$

Step 2: Subtract and then bring the decimal straight down.

$$\begin{array}{r} 9^4 5.^{14} 5^1 0 \\ - \;\; 0. \;\; 7 \;\; 6 \\ \hline 94. \;\; 7 \;\; 4 \end{array}$$

Practice

1. $3.4 - 2.68 =$

2. $69.4 - 5.04 =$

3. $15 - 0.935 =$

4. $0.48 - 0.3925 =$

5. $3.7 - 0.1987 =$

6. $12 - 1.932 =$

7. $0.2 - 0.025 =$

8. $14.47 - 0.3108 =$

9. $87.56 - 0.124 =$

10. $0.07 - 0.007 =$

Applications

1. A patient started with a 1 liter bag of IV solution. When the doctor checked in on the patient, the bag contained 0.35 liters of solution. How much solution was infused into the patient?

2. A bottle of medicine contains 30 milliliters. After withdrawing 2.25 milliliters for an injection, how many milliliters of medicine remain in the bottle?

3. A patient is to receive 4.25 milligrams of a drug daily. The patient has already received 2.75 milligrams. What is his remaining dosage in milligrams?

4. Patient B is on a low fat diet. He weighed 89.9 kilograms last month. This month he weighs 88.45 kilograms. How many kilograms has he lost?

5. A patient had a 101.4°F temperature. If after medication, the patient is at 99.6°F, what is the decrease in the patient's temperature?

Multiplication of Decimals

To multiply decimals, multiply the two numbers using the same process used in whole number multiplication. Do not line up the decimals. The decimals places are counted, not aligned in decimal multiplication.

Example

$$4.75 \times .4$$

Step 1: Write the problem vertically.

$$
\begin{array}{r}
4.75 \\
\times \quad .4 \\
\hline
\end{array}
$$

Step 2: Multiply the numbers.

$$
\begin{array}{r}
4.75 \\
\times \quad .4 \\
\hline
1900
\end{array}
$$

Step 3: Count the number of total decimal places in the two numbers multiplied together. Count these places from the right in to the left. Then begin at the right of the answer and count over the same number of places and place the decimal.

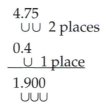

$$
\begin{array}{r}
4.75 \\
\text{UU} \; 2 \text{ places} \\
0.4 \\
\underline{\text{U} \; 1 \text{ place}} \\
1.900 \\
\text{UUU}
\end{array}
$$

Place the decimal point three places from the right since there are three decimal places in the numbers you multiplied. The extra zeros are dropped unless they serve a particular purpose, such as place holders for money in dollar figures.

$$
\begin{array}{rcl}
17.750 & \to & 17.75 \\
205.12600 & \to & 205.126 \\
\$12.00 & \to & \$12.00
\end{array}
$$

Practice   Set up multiplication problems vertically.

1. 4.2×3

2. 9.3×7

3. 21×1.6

4. 465×0.3

5. 9.17×14

6. 0.985×50

7. 6.74×0.12

8. 3.190×0.56

9. 0.278×1.7

10. 4.79×2.2

11. 0.08×0.03

12. 5.6×0.39

13. 5.175×29.2

14. $3{,}764 \times 13.75$

15. 9.708×0.17

16. 114.6×22.6

17. 190.8×0.04

18. 827.9×1.9

19. 574×12.095

20. 0.135×73.7

21. 53.9×24.9

22. 204.7×13.87

23. 0.347×28.95

24. 94.13×32.09

Applications
1. Village Center health care workers' earnings start at $10.52 an hour. If the employees work 40 hours per week, what is the minimum amount that each worker could earn a week?

2. One mile has 1.6 kilometers. How many kilometers are in 35.5 miles?

3. Sheila earns $13.05 an hour. If she works 124 hours in August, what are her gross earnings for the month?

4. One kilogram equals 2.2 pounds. If Patient A weighs 79.5 kilograms, what is his weight in pounds?

5. The recreation department is making placemats. The cost of materials for each placemat is $1.28. The activity director is estimating the cost of ma-

terials for 100 placemats. What is the estimated budget needed for this project?

Division of Decimals

To divide decimals, one needs to place the decimal first, then divide the two numbers. Once the decimal is placed, it is not moved. Students have a tendency to want to move the decimal once the division process is underway; the result is an error in decimal placement.

Follow the steps below to divide a decimal that has a decimal in the dividend:

Step 1: Move the decimal straight up to the same place in the quotient. Place the decimal and then divide the numbers.

$$6\overline{)2.58}$$

Step 2: Divide, adding a zero in front of all decimal numbers that do not include a whole number.

$$
\begin{array}{r}
0.43 \\
6\overline{)2.58} \\
2\ 4 \\
\hline
18 \\
18 \\
\hline
0
\end{array}
$$

Practice

1. $19\overline{)11.97}$

2. $5\overline{)67.75}$

3. $2\overline{)0.464}$

4. $21\overline{)9.03}$

5. $12\overline{)1.44}$

6. $4\overline{)68.4}$

7. $32\overline{)1676.8}$

8. $17\overline{)51.17}$

9. $25\overline{)75.50}$

10. $34\overline{)2603.72}$

Zeros as Placeholders in Decimal Division

Health care students may need some practice in dividing decimals that involve zeros in the quotient. This is one area where common errors are made. To avoid this situation, recall that after a number has been brought down from the dividend, the divisor must be applied to the number. If it cannot, then a zero must be placed in the quotient. Place the decimal and then divide the numbers. Use a zero to hold a space.

Example

$$
\begin{array}{r}
2.405 \\
14\overline{)33.67} \\
28\downarrow \\
\hline
56 \\
56\downarrow \\
\hline
07 \\
0\downarrow \\
\hline
70 \\
70 \\
\hline
0
\end{array}
$$

Because 14 cannot go into 7, place a 0 in the quotient.

Setup Tip

Remember in division problem setup:

$475 \div 4.5 =$

$\longrightarrow \quad 4.5\overline{)475}$

*The last number in the problem divides into the first number.

Practice

1. $530 \div 0.5$

2. $0.081 \div 9$

3. $66.56 \div 32$

4. $0.022 \div 11$

5. $3.297 \div 3$

6. $0.6250 \div 5$

7. $183.96 \div 6$

8. $6.030 \div 3$

9. $0.18891 \div 0.9$

10. $12.24 \div 4$

Simplified Multiplication and Division of Decimals

Using the shortcuts of simplified multiplication and division can save you time in working with decimals. In health care fields, this shortcut is important to your work in metrics and in efficiently working longer problems.

This shortcut only works with multiples of ten: 10, 100, 1,000, etc. The process is straightforward. To multiply, move the decimal to the right. To divide, move the decimal to the left. The number of spaces depends on which multiple you are working with. Look at the number of zeros included in the multiple, then move the decimal in either direction depending on the operation: multiplication or division, the same number of spaces and the number of zeros.

Simplified Multiplication

To multiply by 10, locate the decimal and move it to the right one place.

To multiply by 100, locate the decimal and move it to the right two places.

To multiply by 1,000, locate the decimal and move it to the right three places.

> Whole numbers have their decimal places to the far right of the last digit. 9 = 9., 75 = 75., 125 = 125.

Example

$$4.5 \times 10 = 45 \qquad 4.5$$
$$4.5 = 45 \qquad \underline{\times\ 10}$$
$$\cup \qquad\qquad 45.0 \quad \text{(The zero is dropped.)}$$

Note that the answer is the same if the problem is worked the long way. Sometimes zeros must be added as placeholders.

In simplified multiplication locate the decimal, count the zeros in the divisor and move the decimal the same number of places to the right.

Example Zeros must fill the spaces if needed.

$$34.7 \times 1000 = \underline{\qquad}$$
$$34.7\,0\,0 =$$
$$\cup\cup\cup \rightarrow 34{,}700$$

Practice

1. 13.5×10

2. 4.56×100

3. 125.75×10

4. $1{,}000 \times 45.3$

5. 0.06×100

6. 0.234×10

7. $12.67 \times 1{,}000$

8. 0.975×100

9. $0.476 \times 1{,}000$

10. 87×10

11. 1.345×10

12. $98.345 \times 1{,}000$

13. 1.009×10

14. 32.901×100

15. $23.850 \times 1{,}000$

Simplified Division

To divide by 10, locate the decimal and move it to the left one place.

To divide by 100, locate the decimal and move it to the left two places.

To divide by 1,000, locate the decimal and move it to the left three places.

In simplified division, locate the decimal, count the zeros in the divisor and move the decimal the same number of places to the left.

Example $9.5 \div 10 = $ _____ $0.75 \div 100 = $ _____
              9.5 $0\,0\,0.75 \rightarrow 0.0075$ Zeros must be used to fill
              $\cup \rightarrow 0.95$ $\cup\,\cup$ in places if needed.

Practice   1. $12.9 \div 10$

              2. $45.56 \div 100$

              3. $125 \div 10$

              4. $98.762 \div 1{,}000$

              5. $0.25 \div 10$

              6. $176.5 \div 100$

              7. $15.8 \div 100$

              8. $3{,}234 \div 10$

              9. $32.50 \div 100$

10. $0.09 \div 10$

11. $10{,}010 \div 1{,}000$

12. $9{,}765 \div 1{,}000$

13. $3.076 \div 100$

14. $429.6 \div 1{,}000$

15. $10.275 \div 100$

Applications

1. The nursing student spends $379.50 for textbooks. If the student purchases 6 textbooks, what is the average cost of each book?

2. A patient's goal is to lose 24.6 pounds. The doctor wants the patient to lose these pounds slowly, over a twelve-month period. How many pounds should the patient attempt to lose each month?

3. Doctor Brown prescribed a medication dosage of 4.5 grams. How many 1.5 gram tablets need to be administered?

4. The dietitian serves a protein dish at three meals. If the total daily grams of protein are 225.9 grams, assuming that the grams are equally divided for the three meals a day, what is the average meal's grams of protein?

5. Bob made $131.20 in 5 hours. What is his hourly wage?

Changing Decimals to Fractions

It is important to be able to convert between number systems so that you are comfortable with comparing sizes of items or quantities of supplies. Changing decimals to fractions requires the use of decimal places and placing the numbers in fractions that represent the very same numbers.

Example Convert 0.457 to a fraction.

Step 1: To convert a decimal to a fraction, count the number of decimal places in the decimal number.

$$0.\underline{4}\,\underline{5}\,\underline{7} \qquad \text{three decimal places means}$$
thousandths in decimal numbers.

Step 2: Write the number 457 as the numerator and 1,000 as the denominator.

$$\frac{457}{1{,}000}$$

Step 3: Reduce if necessary. $^{457}/_{1000}$ cannot be reduced. The answer is $^{457}/_{1000}$.

Example Convert 2.75 to a fraction.

Step 1: Place 2 as the whole number. Your answer is going to be a mixed number because there is a whole number. Count the decimal places in .$\underline{7}\,\underline{5}$ = two places.

$$2\,\underline{\qquad}$$

Step 2: Write 75 as the numerator and 100 as the denominator.

$$2\frac{75}{100}$$

Step 3: Reduce the fraction to 2 3/4 because

$$\frac{75}{100} = \frac{\cancel{25} \times 3}{\cancel{25} \times 4} \rightarrow \frac{3}{4}$$

The answer is $2\,^3/_4$.

Practice Convert the decimals to fractions:

1. 0.04

2. 0.025

3. 6.25

4. 1.78

5. 225.05

6. 10.50

7. 7.75

8. 0.08

9. 9.3

10. 100.46

Changing Fractions to Decimals

To change fractions to decimals, divide the denominator into the numerator. Critical to the success of this division is the placement of the decimal. Once it is placed, do not move it.

Example Change $^3/_4$ to a decimal. Divide the denominator into the numerator. Place a decimal after 3 and move it straight up into the quotient. Then add a zero after 3 and divide. Add zeros as needed to continue the division process.

$$
\begin{array}{r}
.75 \\
4\overline{)3.0} \\
28\downarrow \\
\overline{20} \\
20 \\
\overline{0}
\end{array}
$$

Example Change $^1/_3$ into a decimal. Divide 3 into 1. Place the decimal. Add zeros as needed to continue division. The division may not come out evenly, but rather begin to repeat itself. After two places, make the remainder into a fraction by putting the remaining number over the divisor.

$$
\begin{array}{r}
.33^1/_3 \\
3\overline{)1.0} \\
9\downarrow \\
\overline{10} \\
9 \\
\overline{1}
\end{array}
$$

> When the decimal answer is a number like 0.50, drop the final zero so that the answer is 0.5.

Practice
1. $\dfrac{1}{2}$

2. $\dfrac{3}{5}$

3. $\dfrac{7}{8}$

4. $\dfrac{1}{6}$

5. $\dfrac{6}{25}$

6. $\dfrac{5}{12}$

7. $\dfrac{3}{15}$

8. $\dfrac{7}{10}$

9. $\dfrac{5}{6}$

10. $\dfrac{3}{18}$

Temperature Conversions with Decimals

The following temperature conversions include decimals. Round the decimal numbers in temperatures to the nearest tenth place. The temperature conversion used in Unit 3: Fractions, relied on fractions. The same fraction method can be converted into a decimal method. In deciding which method to use, select the method of fractions or decimals based on your strongest skill. Then consistently use that conversion formula.

Decimal Conversion Formula

Memorize these setups:

To convert Celsius to Fahrenheit: °C $\times$ 1.8 + 32 = °F

To convert Fahrenheit to Celsius: °F − 32 ÷ 1.8 = °C

Example   To convert from Celsius to Fahrenheit:

$$41°C = \underline{\quad\quad} °F$$

Step 1: Multiply the Celsius temperature by 1.8. The number 1.8 is the decimal form of ⅘.

$$
\begin{array}{r}
41 \\
\times\, 1.8 \\
\hline
328 \\
41 \\
\hline
73.8
\end{array}
$$

Step 2: Add 32 to the step 1 answer.

$$
\begin{array}{r}
73.8 \\
+\, 32 \\
\hline
105.8
\end{array}
$$

The answer is 105.8°F.

To convert from Fahrenheit to Celsius:

Step 1: Subtract the 32 from the Fahrenheit temperature.

$$
\begin{array}{r}
107.6 \\
-\, 32 \\
\hline
75.6
\end{array}
$$

Step 2: Divide the step 1 answer by 1.8.

$$
\rightarrow 1.8\,\overline{)75.6} \rightarrow
\begin{array}{r}
42. \\
18\,\overline{)756.} \\
72 \\
\hline
36 \\
36 \\
\hline
0
\end{array}
$$

The answer is 42°C.

Practice   1. 34°C = \underline{\quad\quad} °F

2. 46.6°F = \underline{\quad\quad} °C

3. 107°C = \underline{\quad\quad} °F

4. 101.5°F = \underline{\quad\quad} °C

5. 42°C = \underline{\quad\quad} °F

6. 40°F = _____ °C

7. 100.4°F = _____ °C

8. 69°C = _____ °F

9. 12°C = _____ °F

10. 105.8°F = _____ °C

Solving Mixed Fraction and Decimal Problems

Sometimes problems will include both fractions and decimals. The very same processes of solving the problems are still needed; however, the order of handling the parts of the problem may vary. Group the math computations inside the problem to best manage the separate operations.

> If the problem has a complex fraction multiplied by a decimal number, work the complex fraction first. Then complete the decimal multiplication.

Example

$$\frac{\frac{1}{2}}{\frac{1}{5}} \times 2.2 =$$

Step 1:

$$\frac{1}{2} \div \frac{1}{5} \rightarrow \frac{1}{2} \times \frac{5}{1} = \frac{5}{2}$$

Reduce to 2 ½. Make the ½ into .5 so that the multiplication is easy. So by first working the complex fraction, the answer is 2.5.

Step 2: Multiply 2.5 × 2.2.

$$\begin{array}{r} 2.5 \\ \times\ 2.2 \\ \hline 50 \\ 50 \\ \hline 5.50 \end{array}$$

The answer to this mixed problem is 5.5.

> If the problem includes a decimal number, handle the decimals by first multiplying straight across, then complete the process by dividing that answer by the denominator. This allows for the division of decimals only once, and it saves time.

Example

$$\frac{0.25}{0.5} \times 1.5$$

Step 1: Multiply 0.25×1.5.

$$
\begin{array}{r}
0.25 \\
\times\, 1.5 \\
\hline
125 \\
25 \\
\hline
0.375
\end{array}
$$

Step 2: Divide 0.375 by 0.5.

$$0.5\overline{)0.375}$$

$$
\begin{array}{r}
0.75 \\
0.5\overline{)0.375} \\
\underline{0.35} \\
0025 \\
\underline{0025} \\
0
\end{array}
$$

The answer is 0.75.

Practice

1. $\dfrac{1/200}{1/100} \times 4.4$

2. $\dfrac{0.8}{0.64} \times 4.5$

3. $\dfrac{3/4}{1/4} \times 2.5$

4. $\dfrac{0.75}{0.15} \times 1.5$

5. $\dfrac{0.002}{0.125} \times 10.5$

6. $\dfrac{1/12}{1/6} \times 3.6$

7. $\dfrac{0.005}{0.01} \times 15.35$

8. $\dfrac{7\frac{1}{2}}{1\frac{1}{2}} \times 5.4$

DECIMAL SELF-TEST

1. Write in words: 0.045

2. What is the sum of 1.7, 19, 0.25, and 0.8?

3. $17 - 0.075$

4. 4.5×1.009

5. $18.04 \div 0.2$

6. Round to the nearest hundredth: 978.735

7. Order these decimals from largest to smallest: 0.81, 0.080, 0.018, 8.018.

8. 10.009×100.

9. A child receives 0.5 milligrams of a drug 4 times a day. How many milligrams is the child's daily dose?

10. A patient receives 2.25 grams of a medication daily. Tablets come in 0.75 gram dosages. How many tablets does the patient take daily?

11. Convert this decimal to a fraction: 0.125

12. Convert this fraction to a decimal: $\dfrac{13}{50}$

13. Convert this fraction to a decimal: $3\dfrac{5}{8}$

14. Convert 103° Fahrenheit to °Celsius.

15. Solve:

$$\dfrac{0.136}{0.2} \times 2.5$$

Unit 5

Ratio and Proportion

Ratio

A ratio is used to show a relationship between two numbers. These numbers are separated by a colon (:) as in 3:4. Ratios may be presented in three formats that provide the setup for solving proportions.

a. 3:4

b. $\dfrac{3}{4}$

c. 3 is to 4

The relationship can represent something as simple as the 1:3 ratio commonly used to mix frozen juices. We use 1 can of frozen juice concentrate to 3 cans of water. Ratios are fractions that represent a part-to-whole relationship. Ratios are always reduced to their lowest form. Example: 8 hours of sleep to 24 hours in a day

$$8{:}24 \rightarrow \frac{8}{24} \qquad \frac{\cancel{8} \times 1}{\cancel{8} \times 3} = \frac{1}{3}, \text{ so the ratio is 1:3.}$$

Write the following relationships as ratios using a colon. Reduce to the lowest terms, if necessary.

1. 5 days out of 7 days

2. eight teeth out of thirty-two teeth

3. 3 students out of 15 students

4. 16 scalpels to 45 syringes

5. 7 inlays to 14 crowns

Proportion

Proportions can be applied to almost every health care profession in one way or another. In addition to on-the-job applications, proportions provide a simple and quick method for solving many everyday math problems such as measurement conversions, recipe conversions for increasing or decreasing the amounts of ingredients, and map mileage.

Proportions are two or more equivalent ratios or fractions. The terms of the first ratio/fraction have the same relationship of part to whole as the second ratio/fraction.

Example $\dfrac{3}{4} = \dfrac{15}{20}$ or 3 : 4 : : 15 : 20   (: : means =)

Test the two ratios/fractions to see whether they are equivalent by multiplying diagonally.

$4 \times 15 = 60$ and $3 \times 20 = 60$. This is a proportion.

If the two numbers that are diagonal result in the same answer when they are multiplied, you are working with a proportion. Proportions are equivalent fractions. Proportions are powerful tools in health care. You can rely on them for solving a majority of your math conversions and problems. Check to see if the following ratios are proportions:

Are these ratios proportions?

1. 5 : 2 = 4 : 1   _____ Yes   _____ No

2. 16 : 15 = 8 : 7   _____ Yes   _____ No

3. 40 : 30 = 4 : 3   _____ Yes   _____ No

4. 10 : 16 = 5 : 8   _____ Yes   _____ No

5. 100 : 1 = 50 : 2   _____ Yes   _____ No

Solving for x

The ratio and proportion method of solving for x is done in two steps.

Step 1: Set the problems up like fractions. If units of measure such as inches and feet are given, place inches across from inches and feet across from feet. Then cross-multiply (diagonally) the two numbers. Set the ratios up like fractions using a vertical line.

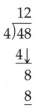
$3 \times 16 = 48$

Step 2: Divide the answer from step 1 by the remaining number.

$$\begin{array}{r} 12 \\ 4\overline{)48} \\ \underline{4\downarrow} \\ 8 \\ \underline{8} \end{array}$$

The answer 12 is the answer to ? or x. This method is an easy way to find the answers for measurement conversions, dosage conversions, and math questions that provide part but not all of the information.

Practice   Solve for x or ?.

1. $20 : 40 = x : 15$

2. $x : 1 = 5 : 10$

3. $4 : 8 = 8 : x$

4. $7 : x = 21 : 24$

5. $3 : 9 = ? : 81$

6. $13 : 39 = 1 : ?$

7. $2 : 11 = ? : 77$

8. $x : 125 = 5 : 25$

9. $2 : 26 = 4 : ?$

10. $1 : x = 5 : 200$

Using ratios is often the simplest method of solving other health care math problems, such as dosage calculations and measurement problems.

Example   Zoe weighs 35 pounds. The doctor ordered a drug that relies on milligrams of medication to kilograms. The pharmacy technician will need to convert pounds to kilograms. By using the ratio of 1 kg to 2.2 pounds, the answer is quickly computed.

$$\frac{known}{} \qquad \frac{unknown}{}$$

$$\frac{1 \text{ kilograms}}{2.2 \text{ pounds}} \qquad \frac{?}{35 \text{ pounds}}$$

Step 1: Multiply the numbers diagonally.

$$1 \times 35 = 35$$

Step 2: Divide 35 by 2.2. The answer is 15.9 kilograms.

So 35 pounds equals 15.9 kilograms.

Example   How many pounds are in 24 ounces?

Set the problem up by placing what you know on the left side of the equation and what you do not know on the right. If you set up all your problems with the known on the left and the unknown on the right, you will have less information for the brain to process because the pattern will be familiar to you.

$$\frac{known}{} \qquad \frac{unknown}{}$$

$$\frac{1 \text{ pound}}{16 \text{ ounces}} \qquad \frac{? \text{ pounds}}{24 \text{ ounces}}$$

Step 1: $1 \times 24 = 24$

Step 2: $24 \div 16 = 1.5$

The answer is 1½ pounds or 1.5 pounds.
An answer for a ratio may have a decimal or a fraction in it.

Example   Bob is 176 centimeters (cm) tall. How tall is he in inches? Round the answer to the nearest tenth.

$$\frac{known}{} \qquad \frac{unknown}{}$$

$$\frac{1 \text{ inch}}{2.54 \text{ cm}} \qquad \frac{? \text{ inches}}{176 \text{ cm}}$$

Step 1: $1 \times 176 = 176$

Step 2: $176 \div 2.54 = 69.29$
Rounded to the nearest tenth.

The answer is 69.3.

$$
\begin{array}{r}
69.29 \\
254.\overline{)17600.} \\
1524\downarrow \\
2360 \\
2286\downarrow \\
740 \\
508\downarrow \\
2320 \\
2286 \\
\hline
34
\end{array}
$$

> Some basic guidelines need to be followed for formatting answers in measurement conversions:
>
> If the answer is in feet, yards, cups, pints, quarts, gallons, teaspoons, tablespoons, or pounds, use fractions if there is a remainder.
>
> If the answer is in kilograms, milliliters, or money amounts, use decimals. The correct format ensures correct answers.

> **Approximate Equivalents**
>
> | 1 inch | = 2.54 centimeters | 1 cup | = 8 ounces |
> |---|---|---|---|
> | 1 foot | = 12 inches | 1 pint | = 500 milliliters |
> | 1 yard | = 3 feet | 1 quart | = 32 ounces |
> | 1 pound | = 16 ounces | 1 quart | = 1,000 milliliters |
> | 1 kilogram | = 2.2 pounds | | |
> | 1 tablespoon | = 3 teaspoons | 1 fluid ounce | = 30 milliliters |
> | 1 quart | = 2 pints | 1 teaspoon | = 5 milliliters |
> | 1 gallon | = 4 quarts | 1 fluid ounce | = 2 tablespoons |
>
> Notice that the conversions are set up so that the 1 elements are all on the left and that these will be placed on the top of the known part of the ratio and proportion equation. This simplifies the learning process, expedites learning, and helps recall of these conversions.

Practice   Because inches are rounded to the nearest tenth, go to the hundredth place and then stop multiplying. At that point, you will have enough information to round to the nearest tenth.

Using this ratio and proportion setup, solve these conversions.

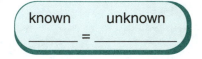

known   unknown
_____ = _____

Set these conversions up using ratios and proportions.

1. 23 feet = _____ yards → $\dfrac{1 \text{ yd}}{3 \text{ ft}} = \dfrac{?}{23 \text{ ft}}$

2. 12 quarts = _____ gallons

3. 4 quarts = _____ pints

4. 4 pints = _____ cups

5. 3 tablespoons = _____ teaspoons

6. 2½ quarts = _____ milliliters

7. ½ cup = _____ ounces

8. 1 injection at $29.50 = 3 injections at _____

9. 3½ pounds = _____ ounces

10. 3 medicine cups = _____ milliliters
(One medicine cup equals 1 fluid ounce)

11. 12.5 mL = _____ teaspoons

12. 5 fluid ounces = _____ tablespoons

13. _____ tablespoons = 15 teaspoons

14. 64 ounces = _____ cups

15. 750 milliliters = _____ pints

16. 48 inches = _____ feet

17. 5 pounds = _____ ounces

18. _____ quarts = 5,000 milliliters

19. _____ kilograms = 11 pounds

20. 3½ cups = _____ ounces

More practice with conversions of measurements between systems and with multiple steps in conversions will be given in Unit 7: Combined Applications.

Word Problems Using Proportions

When doing word problems involving proportions, follow these two basic steps:

Step 1: Set the problem up so that the same type of elements are directly across from one another.

Example   If 12 eggs cost $1.49, how much do 18 eggs cost?

$$\frac{\text{Eggs}}{\text{Cost}} = \frac{\text{Eggs}}{\text{Cost}} \rightarrow \frac{12 \text{ eggs}}{\$1.49} = \frac{18 \text{ eggs}}{\$?}$$

Step 2: Ensure that the story problem is understood, then place the known information on the left side of the proportion and the unknown on the right. By doing so, you will not switch the ratio relationships, but rather rely on the known part to whole relationships.

1. A caplet contains 325 milligrams of medication. How many caplets contain 975 milligrams of medication?

2. If a dose of 100 milligrams is contained in 4 cubic centimeters, how many cubic centimeters are in 40 milligrams?

3. If 35 grams of pure drug are contained in 150 milliliters, how many grams are contained in 75 milliliters?

4. Two tablets of ulcer medication contain 350 milligrams of medication. How many milligrams are in twelve tablets?

5. If 1 kilogram equals 2.2 pounds, how many kilograms are in 61.6 pounds?

Solving for x in More Complex Problems Using Proportion

Decimals and fractions may appear in your proportion problems. Although the numbers may be visually distracting, the *very* same principles apply.

Example $0.25 \text{ mg} : 0.8 \text{ mL} = 0.125 \text{ mg} : x \text{ mL}$

Step 1: Place mg across from mg and mL across from mL. Place the known information on the left side of the equation and the unknown on the right.

known   *unknown*

$\dfrac{0.25 \text{ mg}}{0.8 \text{ mL}}$ $\dfrac{0.125 \text{ mg}}{x \text{ mL}}$

Cross multiply $0.8 \times 0.125 \text{ mg} = 0.1$.

Step 2: $0.1 \div 0.25 = 0.4 \text{ mL}$

Example $\dfrac{1}{8} : \dfrac{1}{2} :: 1 : x$ (:: means =)

Step 1: Set up and cross multiply. Multiply $\frac{1}{2} \times 1 = \frac{1}{2}$.

$$\dfrac{1/8}{1/2} = \dfrac{1}{x}$$

Step 2: Divide $\frac{1}{2}$ by $\frac{1}{8}$.

$$\frac{1}{2} \div \frac{1}{8} \rightarrow \frac{1}{2} \times \frac{8}{1} = \frac{8}{2}, \text{ which is reduced to } 4.$$

Sometimes you will find that medical dosages have both fractions and decimals in the problems. Analyze the situation and convert the numbers into the same system. As a general rule, fractions are always more accurate for calculating than decimals because some decimal numbers have repeating digits, which create variable answers.

Example $\dfrac{1}{16} : 1.6 :: \dfrac{1}{8} x$

Step 1: Convert 1.6 into a fraction. So $1.6 = 1^6/_{10}$. Then multiply $1^6/_{10} \times \frac{1}{8} = {}^2/_{10}$

$$\dfrac{1/16}{1^6/_{10}} = \dfrac{1/8}{x} \qquad 1\frac{6}{10} \times \frac{1}{8} = \frac{16}{10} \times \frac{1}{8} = \frac{16}{80} \text{ or } \frac{2}{10}$$

Step 2: Divide $^2/_{10}$ by $^1/_{16}$.

$$\frac{2}{10} \div \frac{1}{16} \rightarrow \frac{2}{10} \times \frac{16}{1} = \frac{32}{10} \qquad \text{Reduced to } 3^2/_{10} \rightarrow 3^1/_5.$$

Practice   Include a unit of measure in your answer. Round any partial unit to the nearest tenth.

> Tablets can be divided if they are scored; use ½ not 0.5

1. 1.5 mg : 2 caps = 4.5 mg : x caps

2. 8 mg : 2.5 mL = 4 mg : x mL

3. 12.5 mg : 5 mL = 24 mg : x mL

4. 0.3 mg : 1 tab = 6 mg : x tab

5. grains ¼ : 15 mg = grains ? : 60 mg

6. x mg : 0.5 tab = 6 mg : 4 tab

7. grains $^1/_{100}$: 2 mL = grains $^1/_{150}$: x mL

8. 600 mg : 1 cap = x mg : 2 cap

9. 1000 U : 1 mL = 2400 U : x mL

10. 1 tab : 0.1 mg = x tab : 0.15 mg

11. A drug comes in 100 mg tablets. If the doctor orders 150 mg daily, how many tablets should the patient receive daily?

12. A medical chart states that the patient weighs 78.4 kg. What is the patient's weight in pounds? Round to the nearest tenth.

Nutritional Application of Proportions

Carbohydrates, fats, and protein provide fuel factors for our bodies. The factors are easily applied by using proportions to solve for the unknown.

> Carbohydrates → 4 calories per 1 gram
> Fats   → 9 calories per 1 gram
> Proteins   → 4 calories per 1 gram

Example   400 carbohydrate calories = _____ grams

$$\frac{\text{known}}{1 \text{ gram}} \qquad \frac{\text{unknown}}{? \text{ grams}}$$

$$\frac{1 \text{ gram}}{4 \text{ calories}} \qquad \frac{? \text{ grams}}{400 \text{ calories}}$$

Step 1: Multiply diagonally.

$$1 \times 400 = 400$$

Step 2: Divide answer from step 1 (400) by the remaining number in the equation (4).

$$\begin{array}{r} 100 \\ 4\overline{)400} \\ \underline{4} \\ 00 \end{array}$$

So 400 carbohydrate calories are available in 100 grams of carbohydrates.

Use proportion to solve the following problems:

1. 81 calories of fat = _____ grams

2. 120 calories of protein = _____ grams

3. 36 calories of carbohydrate = _____ grams

4. 145 calories of carbohydrate = _____ grams

5. _____ calories in 12 grams of protein

6. _____ calories in 99 grams of fat

7. _____ calories in 328 grams of carbohydrate

8. _____ calories in 2450 grams of protein

Proportion is also useful in solving measurement problems that have to do with amounts of sodium, calories, fat, and protein in food or an amount in a drug dosage. The proportion will use the information in a scenario to solve for the unknown quantities in a specific amount.

Example If one glass of milk contains 280 milligrams of calcium, how much calcium is in 1½ glasses of milk?

$$\frac{1 \text{ glass}}{280 \text{ mg}} = \frac{1\frac{1}{2} \text{ glasses}}{? \text{ mg}}$$

$$280 \times 1\frac{1}{2} = 420 \text{ mg of calcium}$$

1. One-half cup of baked beans contains 430 mg of sodium. How many milligrams of sodium are there in ¾ cup of baked beans?

2. Baked beans contain 33 grams of carbohydrates in a ½ cup serving. How many milligrams of carbohydrates are in three ½ cup servings?

3. A ½ cup serving of fruit cocktail contains 55 milligrams of potassium. How many milligrams of potassium are in 2 cups of fruit cocktail?

4. If ½ cup of fruit cocktail contains 13 grams of sugar, then 1¼ cup of fruit cocktail contains how many grams of sugar?

5. Old-fashioned oatmeal contains 27 grams of carbohydrates per ½ cup of dry oats. How many grams of carbohydrate are available in 2 ¼ cups of the dry oats?

RATIO AND PROPORTION SELF-TEST

Show all your work.

1. Write a definition for proportion. Provide one health profession application or example.

2. 30 : 120 = ? : 12

3. 1 glass contains 8 ounces. How many full glasses are in 78 ounces?

4. $\frac{1}{2} : 4 = \frac{1}{3} : x$

5. $x : 625 = 1 : 5$

6. If 10 milligrams are contained in 2 milliliters, how many milligrams are contained in 28 milliliters?

7. A tablet contains 30 mg of medication. How many tablets will be needed to provide Ms. Smith with 240 mg of medication?

8. 100 mcg of a drug are contained in 2 cc. How many cc are contained in 15 mcg?

9. $\frac{1}{100} : 6 = ? : 8$

10. $0.04 : 0.5 = 0.12 : ?$

11. How many minutes are in 130 seconds? Your answer will have both minutes and seconds. Show your setup.

12. Four out of every six dental patients request fluoride treatment after their dental cleaning treatments. If 120 patients have dental cleanings this week, how many will choose to have fluoride treatments as well?

13. If the doctor's office uses 128 disposal thermometer covers each day, how many covers will be used in a five-day workweek?

14. Solve: $\dfrac{1}{125}$:   3 : : _____ : 12

15. If the doctor ordered six ounces of cranberry juice four times a day for four days, how many total ounces would be served the patient?

Unit 6

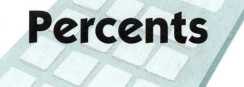

Percents are another example of a part-to-whole relationship in math. Percents are parts of one hundred and appear as 35%. Percents can be written as fractions: 35 parts of 100 or $^{35}/_{100}$.

Knowledge of percents in health care will help you understand the strength in percent of solutions for patient medications, interest on loans and taxes, and discounts and markups in pharmacies and retail stores. In general, percent applications are seen less frequently than fractions and decimals by general health care professionals.

Percent-to-Decimal Conversion

To convert a percent to a decimal, shift the decimal point two places to the left. The process of doing this quick division replaces having to divide the number by 100. This is the same method of simplified division as was shown in Unit 4: Decimals.

> A whole number has its decimal to the far right of the final digit or number.
>
> $$125\% = 125.\% \qquad 76\% = 76.\%$$

Example
$$75\% \rightarrow 7\ 5.\ \% \rightarrow 0.75$$
$$\cup\ \cup$$

If a percent has a fractional part, the decimal occurs between the whole number and the fractional part.

93

Example $33\frac{1}{3}\% \rightarrow 33.\frac{1}{3}\% \rightarrow 0.33\frac{1}{3}$

Practice Convert from percents to decimals:

1. 45%

2. 57%

3. 78⅓%

4. 101%

5. 44½%

Decimal-to-Percent Conversion

To convert a decimal to a percent, shift the decimal point two places to the right. This is the simplified multiplication method as practiced in Unit 4: Decimals.

If a number has a decimal in it and you are converting from a decimal to a percent, use the existing decimal point as the starting point for the conversion. It is possible to have percents greater than 100.

> Begin counting from wherever the decimal is placed.
>
> $0.023 \rightarrow 02.3\%$ $2.56 \rightarrow 256\%$
>
> Handle a mixed fraction by placing the decimal point between whole number and the fraction, then convert the fraction to a whole number by dividing the numerator by the denominator. Then move the decimal two places right and add a % sign.
>
> $14\frac{3}{4} \rightarrow 1475\%$

Examples $0.25 \rightarrow 0.2\ 5\% = 25\%$
$\qquad\qquad\qquad\qquad \cup\ \cup$
$\qquad\qquad 13 \rightarrow 13. \rightarrow 13.0\ 0\% = 1300\%$
$\qquad\qquad\qquad\qquad\qquad \cup\ \cup$

Practice Convert from decimals to percents:

1. 0.625

2. 55.75

3. 8.6

4. 12.5

5. 0.076

Mixed Practice   1. 76.89% to a decimal

2. 0.05% to a decimal

3. 86% to a decimal

4. 6.25% to a percent

5. 0.078 to a percent

6. 9¾ to a percent

7. 1.25¼ to a percent

8. 78⅛% to a decimal

9. 1.5% to a decimal

10. 0.67¼ to a percent

Using Proportion to Solve Percent Problems

Proportions are also very useful in solving percent problems. To accomplish this, use the formula:

$$\frac{\%}{100} = \frac{\text{is (the part)}}{\text{whole (the total)}}$$

To solve any percent problem, take the information from the problem and put it into the formula. There are three possible places that the information can go.

$$\frac{?}{100} = \frac{?}{?}$$

The 100 never changes because that indicates that every percent is part of 100. It is important to set up the problem correctly. The following questions ask for different information. Therefore, the setup of the problems will be different.

Problem	**Setup**
What is 25% of 75?	$\dfrac{25}{100} = \dfrac{?}{75}$
What % of 75 is 18.75?	$\dfrac{?}{100} = \dfrac{18.75}{75}$
18.75 is 25% of what?	$\dfrac{25}{100} = \dfrac{18.75}{?}$

Note that the ? is in a different place each time. When the problem is worked, each of the above answers will be different.

Practice   Set up the problems, but do not solve.

   1. What is 25% of 200?

   2. 75 is what % of 125?

   3. Find 8.5% of 224.

   4. 40 percent of what number is 350?

   5. 18 is what percent of 150?

   6. What is 1½% of 400?

   7. 75 of 90 is what percent?

   8. Out of 200, 140 is what percent?

   9. 50% of what number is 75?

   10. 8⅓% of 144 is what?

To solve percent problems in health care, one needs to be aware that the problem may include whole numbers, fractions, and decimals. The skills used in percents draw on the foundation you have in these areas of math computation. It is important to remember and apply the fraction concepts learned when dealing with fractions in percents because a fraction is more accurate and exact than a decimal number that has a repeating final digit.

To solve percent problems, use the proportion method studied in Unit 5: Ratio and Proportion.

Example   15 is what percent of 300?

$$\frac{x\%}{100} = \frac{15}{300}$$

Step 1: Cross multiply the two numbers on the diagonal.

$$(100 \times 15 = 1500)$$

Step 2: Divide the step 1 answer by the remaining number—the one diagonal from the x or ?

$$1{,}500 \div 300 = 5$$

The answer is 5%. So we know that 15 is 5% of 300.

Practice   1. 15% of 120 is _____.

   2. 33 is what % of 44?

3. 62 is what percent of 248?

4. 40% of 120 is what?

5. What is 35% of 16.8?

6. Find 9% of 3,090.

7. 45 is what percent of 200?

8. 74 is what percent of 74?

9. What is 44% of 40?

10. 121 is what % of 220?

More complex percents include fractions, and the most efficient way of handling these is as complex fractions. By setting up the problem in proportion format, the work is put into manageable steps. A common error is that students multiply the first two numbers and consider their work done; however, there is always a final division step that must be performed.

Example   What is 8⅓% of 150?

$$\frac{8^{1}/_{3}}{100} = \frac{x}{150}$$

Step 1: Multiply 8⅓ and 150. Deal with the fraction; do not change it to a decimal because if you do, your answer will not be as exact. Convert the mixed fraction into an improper fraction. Multiply the whole number by the denominator and add the numerator. Place this number over the denominator. Then multiply this improper fraction by the number 150.

$$8^{1}/_{3} = \frac{25}{3} \times 150 = \frac{3,750}{3} = 1250$$

Step 2: Divide the step 1 answer of 1,250 by 100. Use simplified division. Simplified division moves the decimal 2 places to the left to divide by 100.

$$1,250 \rightarrow 1,2\,5\,0 \ \underset{\cup\cup}{} = 12.5 \text{ or } 12^{1}/_{2} \qquad 0.5 \text{ equals } {}^{1}/_{2}.$$

Practice

1. What is 33⅓% of 125? Round to the nearest hundredth.

2. 1½% of 400 is what?

3. 66⅔% of 90 is what?

4. 35¼% is what part of 150? Round to the nearest hundredth.

5. 12½% of 125 is what? Round to the nearest hundredth.

6. 50 is 83⅓% of what number?

7. 160 is 12½% of what number?

8. 45 is 15⅓% of what number? Round to the nearest hundredth.

9. 200 is 37½% of what number? Round to the nearest hundredth.

10. 87½% of 120 is what?

Two other applications of percents are important for the health care student: the percent strength of a solution and the single trade discount.

Percent Strength of Solutions

The strength of solutions is an important application of percents. A solution is a liquid that has had medication, minerals, or other products dissolved in it. Percent strength refers to how much of a substance has been dissolved in a specific amount of liquid.

Key to percent strength is your knowledge of part-to-whole relationships: A percent is x parts to 100 total parts. Solution refers to a two-part substance: a solute that is the drug, mineral, or product and a solvent or liquid that can be a variety depending on the medical application. Solutes will occur either as a dry drug measured in grams or as a liquid measured in milliliters. The total volume of the liquid is always in milliliters.

Example   A 15% drug solution has 15 parts of drug to 100 parts of solution. There are 15 grams of drug to 100 milliliters of solution. As a ratio, this would be shown in the reduced form as 3:20.

Sometimes the solution will be given as a ratio rather than a percent. To express the solution strength as a percent, set up the problem as a proportion with 100 ml the total solution. Recall that percent is always part of 100.

Practice   Percent strength: What is the ratio of pure drug to solution?

1. 4% solution   _____

2. 10% solution   _____

3. 1½% solution   _____

4. 7.5% solution   _____

5. 5% solution   _____

Knowledge of proportion is useful in converting to smaller or larger amounts of solution. In health care, professionals may not always require 100 mL of a solution. We must be able to maintain the correct ratio of pure drug to solution to ensure that the patient is getting the medication or solution the doctor intended. It is important to note that the ratio of pure drug remains consistent no matter how much solution is to be prepared.

Example   Percent strength 8% means that there are 8 grams of drug to 100 ml of solution. If the doctor orders 25 ml of an 8% strength solution, then a proportion may be used to ensure that the ratio of pure drug to solution represents 8%.

$$\underset{\text{100 mL solution}}{\overset{\text{8 grams of drugs}}{\underbrace{}}} = \underset{\text{25 mL solution}}{\overset{\text{? grams of drug}}{\underbrace{}}}$$

known   *unknown*
$$\frac{\text{8 grams of drugs}}{\text{100 mL solution}} = \frac{\text{? grams of drug}}{\text{25 mL solution}}$$

Step 1: $8 \times 25 = 200$

Step 2: $200 \div 100 = 2$

So to make 25 mL of an 8% solution using this ratio of pure drug to solution, 2 grams of pure drug to 25 mL of solution are required. This keeps the percent strength of the medication consistent with the doctor's order for an 8% strength solution. Note that the amount of mixed solution changes, not the percent strength itself.

Example 10 grams of drug in 25 milliliters of solution. What is the percent strength of this medication?

To convert this ratio into a percent, write it as a proportion. Then solve for x which will become the percent.

$$\overset{known}{\frac{10 \text{ grams}}{25 \text{ grams}}} = \overset{unknown}{\frac{x}{100 \text{ mL}}}$$

Follow proportion steps to solve. Cross multiply $10 \times 100 = 1{,}000$. Divide 1,000 by 25 = 40, so the answer is 40% strength.

Practice 1. The doctor has ordered a 5% saline solution to be prepared. How many grams of pure drug will be needed to make each of these amounts of solution at the 5% strength?

a. 25 mL of solution

b. 35 mL of solution

c. 65 mL of solution

d. 125 mL of solution

2. 9 mL of pure drug are in 100 ml of solution.

a. What is the percent strength of the solution?

b. How many milliliters of drug are in 75 mL of that solution?

3. 15 grams of pure drug are in 50 mL.

    a. What is the percent strength of the solution?

    b. How many grams of pure drug are in 200 mL of the solution?

Single Trade Discount

Single trade discounts are useful to individuals who handle products or inventory that must be marked up. The single trade discount provides the net price of items when a single discount has been given. Some health care organizations that use certain name brands receive these discounts from manufacturers of the products they use or sell most often.

Example What is the net price of a surgical instrument listed at $189.90 with a trade discount of 40%?

Step 1: The percentage is first made into a decimal by moving the decimal point two places to the left. Then, multiply the list price by the trade discount.

> You may need to round your decimal number to the nearest cent.

$$
\begin{array}{r}
\$189.90 \\
\times \quad .40 \\
\hline
00000 \\
75960 \\
\hline
\$75.96
\end{array}
$$

Step 2: Subtract the amount of the discount (the answer from step 1) from the list price to get the net price.

$$
\begin{array}{r}
\$189.90 \\
-75.96 \\
\hline
\$113.94
\end{array}
$$

The net price of this instrument is $113.94.

Practice Find the net price by using the single trade discount method. If necessary, round to the nearest penny. Show your work.

	List Price	Trade Discount	Amount of Discount	Net Price
1.	$475.50	15%	_____	_____
2.	$179.85	20%	_____	_____
3.	$125.55	12.5%	_____	_____
4.	$455.86	30%	_____	_____
5.	$352.90	25%	_____	_____
6.	$72.35	10%	_____	_____
7.	$250.40	45%	_____	_____
8.	$862.75	35%	_____	_____
9.	$158.00	40%	_____	_____
10.	$73.85	10%	_____	_____

PERCENT SELF-TEST

1. Write the definition of a percent. Provide one example.

2. Convert the following into percents:

   a. $0.87\frac{1}{4}$

   b. $\dfrac{5}{6}$

3. 75% of 325 is what number?

4. 8 is what % of 40?

5. 28 is 14% of what number?

6. What does 5½% solution mean?

7. The doctor has ordered 25 ml of 9% saline solution. How much pure drug is needed to make this order?

8. The list price for a case of medicine is $129.50. Your pharmacy will receive a 12% trade discount.

   a. What is the amount of the discount? _____

   b. What is the net case cost of the medicine? _____

9. What percent is 3 tablets of a prescription written for 36 tablets?

10. If a pharmacy gave a 15% discount on walkers, what would be the discount for a total bill of $326.00 for a six-month rental?

11. If a ratio of 3 : 25 is given for a solution, what percent strength is this solution?

12. What is ½% of 500?

13. Express 8 : 125 as a percent.

14. What is ¾% of 20?

15. 35 is 0.05% of what?

Unit 7

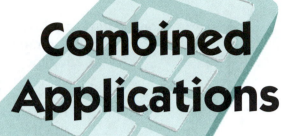

Combined Applications

Health care workers rely on a variety of math systems to achieve their daily tasks. Knowledge of ways to convert efficiently between systems will benefit you on the job as your expertise grows and your circle of responsibility increases. It is important to have the ability to convert between fractions, decimals, ratios, and percents. Although these skills have been separately reviewed, they are brought together here to develop some strategies for doing these conversions in the most efficient way.

Conversions among Fractions, Decimals, Ratios, and Percent

Review the basics of conversion:

Conversion	Method/Formula
Fraction to decimal	Divide the denominator into the numerator.

$$\frac{3}{4} = \begin{array}{r} 0.75 \\ 4\overline{)3.0} \\ \underline{28}\downarrow \\ 20 \\ \underline{20} \\ 0 \end{array}$$

Decimal to fraction	Count the decimal places, place the number over 1 with zeros to match the same number of decimal places.

$$0.0\underline{2}\ (2\ \text{places}) \rightarrow 2/1\underline{0}\,\underline{0}\ (2\ \text{zeros})$$

Reduce to $^1/_{50}$.

Proper fraction to ratio, ratio to proper fraction	Ratios are shown with : instead of /. Fractions and ratios are interchangeable simply by changing the symbol.

$$^1/_8 \rightarrow 1:8 \quad \text{and} \quad 4:31 \rightarrow {}^4/_{31}$$

The first ratio number is always the numerator and the second ratio number is always the denominator. All fractions and ratios must be in lowest terms.

Mixed number to ratio to mixed number	If the fraction is a mixed number, the mixed ratio number must first be made into an improper fraction before setting up the ratio.

$$1^3/_4 \rightarrow 1 \times 4 + 3 = {}^7/_4 \rightarrow 7:4$$

If the ratio is an improper fraction when the conversion is made, make it a mixed number.

$$^{11}/_4 \rightarrow 11 \div 4 = 2^3/_4$$

Decimal to percent	Move the decimal point two places to the right. Add the percent sign.

$$0.25 \rightarrow 25\% \qquad 1.456 \rightarrow 145.6\%$$

Percent to decimal	Move the decimal point two places to the left. Add zeros if needed as placeholders.

$$90\% \rightarrow 0.9 \quad \text{and} \quad 5\% \rightarrow 0.05$$
$$57^1/_2\% \rightarrow 0.57^1/_2 \text{ or } 0.575$$

Fraction to percent	Convert fraction to decimal, then to percent.

Decimal or percent to ratio	Convert to fraction, then change sign to ratio.

Convert the following numbers to the other number systems. Using the review sheet of conversion methods, try to compute only one math problem per line by carefully selecting the order of the conversions to be done. By carefully selecting the order of conversions, you will minimize extra work.

Example	**Fraction**	**Decimal**	**Ratio**	**Percent**
	_____	0.05	_____	_____

Figuring out the order takes a little practice. When 0.05 is changed to a percent first, no math calculation needs to be done: Simply move the decimal.

Fraction	Decimal	Ratio	Percent
_____	0.05	_____	5%

Next convert the decimal to a fraction. Count the number of decimal places and then place the 5 over a 1 with the same number of zeros as the decimal places. Reduce the fraction to lowest terms.

Fraction	Decimal	Ratio	Percent
$5/100 \rightarrow 1/20$	0.05	_____	5%

Take the reduced fraction and write it in ratio form.

Fraction	Decimal	Ratio	Percent
$5/100 \rightarrow 1/20$	0.05	1 : 20	5%

Example

Fraction	Decimal	Ratio	Percent
$7^3/_5$	_____	_____	_____

This mixed number must be made into an improper fraction before it can become a ratio.

$$(7 \times 5 + 3 = 38 \rightarrow {}^{38}/_5)$$

Change the signs from / to : to make the ratio.

Fraction	Decimal	Ratio	Percent
$7^3/_5$	_____	38 : 5	_____

Next change to a decimal. Handle the whole number 7 separately. Place it on the line as a whole number, then divide the denominator into the numerator.

$$3 \div 5 = 0.6$$

Add this to the whole number to make 7.6.

Fraction	Decimal	Ratio	Percent
$7^3/_5$	7.6	38 : 5	_____

Finally, move the decimal point from the decimal number two places to the right. Add the percent sign.

Fraction	Decimal	Ratio	Percent
$7\frac{3}{5}$	7.6	38 : 5	760%

Suggested Order of Operations

If starting with percent, move from → decimal → fraction → ratio.

If starting with ratio, move from → fraction → decimal → percent.

If starting with fraction, move from → ratio → decimal → percent.

If starting with decimal, move from → percent → fraction → ratio.

Some conversions can be memorized easily:

½ → 0.5 → 50%

¼ → 0.25 → 25%

¾ → 0.75 → 75%

⅓ → 0.33⅓ → 33⅓%

⅔ → 0.66⅔ → 66⅔%

Provide the following measures. Reduce to lowest terms as necessary. Round to the nearest hundredth, if necessary.

	Fraction	Decimal	Ratio	Percent
1.	¾	_____	_____	_____
2.	_____	_____	1 : 20	_____
3.	_____	_____	_____	50%
4.	_____	0.625	_____	_____
5.	_____	_____	1 : 250	_____
6.	⅞	_____	_____	_____
7.	_____	0.06	_____	_____
8.	_____	_____	_____	12.5%
9.	⅒	_____	_____	_____
10.	_____	_____	_____	33⅓%
11.	_____	1.36	_____	_____
12.	12½	_____	_____	_____

	Fraction	Decimal	Ratio	Percent
13.	_____	_____	2 : 5	_____
14.	_____	0.66⅔	_____	_____
15.	_____	_____	16 : 25	_____
16.	_____	0.004	_____	_____
17.	⅝	_____	_____	_____
18.	_____	_____	_____	7¼%
19.	_____	0.01	_____	_____

Using Combined Applications in Measurement Conversion

In health care, a solid working knowledge of weights and measures is essential. Three systems of measure will be used in your work: household or standard measurements and metric measurement, covered in this unit, and apothecary measurement, covered in Unit 8: Dosage Calculations. Critical to your success in measurement conversion is your ability to remember a few key conversions and the proportion method for solving conversions. Metric-to-metric conversions use a different conversion method, which is also covered in Unit 8.

Household or standard measurements are used by all of us in our daily activities. Household measures tend to be less accurate than either metric or apothecary because of their nature and our methods of measuring them. So household measures are used in the less critical measurements in health care. Abbreviations are used and some new abbreviations are introduced below:

Drop = gtt

Teaspoon = t (tsp)

Tablespoon = T (tbsp)

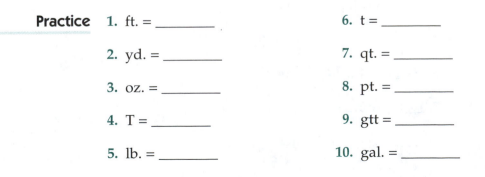

Practice

1. ft. = _____

2. yd. = _____

3. oz. = _____

4. T = _____

5. lb. = _____

6. t = _____

7. qt. = _____

8. pt. = _____

9. gtt = _____

10. gal. = _____

Standard Units of Measure

The basics of standard measure conversion were covered in Unit 5: Ratio and Proportion. To refresh yourself on the proportion application to measurement conversions, complete the review exercises.

Time		Approximate Equivalents	
1 minute	= 60 seconds	grain 1	= 60 milligrams
1 day	= 24 hours	1 teaspoon	= 5 milliliters
1 week	= 7 days	1 tablespoon	= 3 teaspoons
1 year	= 12 months	fluid dram 1	= 4 milliliters
Weight		fluid ounce 1	= fluidrams 8
		fluid ounce 1	= 2 tablespoons
1 kilogram	= 2.2 pounds	fluid ounce 1	= 30 milliliters
1 pound	= 16 ounces	1 cup	= 250 milliliters
Linear Measure			= fluid ounces 8
1 foot	= 12 inches	1 pint	= 500 milliliters
1 yard	= 3 feet		= 2 cups or fluid ounces 16
1 meter	= 39.4 inches		
1 inch	= 2.5 or 2.54 centimeters	1 quart	= fluid ounces 32
			= 1 liter or 1000 mL
Liquid Measure		1 cubic centimeter	= 1 milliliter
1 tablespoon	= 3 teaspoons	1 kilogram	= 2.2 pounds
1 cup	= 8 ounces		
1 pint	= 2 cups	fluid ounce 1	= 2 tablespoons
1 quart	= 2 pints		
1 gallon	= 4 quarts		

Review   Use the provided tables to assist you in using proportions.

1. 1,250 ml = _____ pints

2. 15 kilograms = _____ pounds

3. 12.5 inches = _____ centimeters

4. _____ milliliters = 13 teaspoons

5. _____ ounces = 90 milliliters

6. 38.1 centimeters = _ inches

7. _____ ounces = 1½ pints

8. _____ quarts = 15 liters

9. _____ teaspoons = 12.5 milliliters

10. _____ cubic centimeters = 15 teaspoons

More Combined Applications

Sometimes measurement conversions require more than one conversion to get to the answer.

Example Two conversions are required to convert from ounces to teaspoons:

Step 1: Convert the ounces to milliliters:

$$\overset{known}{\frac{1 \text{ ounce}}{20 \text{ milliliters}}} = \overset{unknown}{\frac{8 \text{ ounces}}{? \text{ milliliters}}} \rightarrow 160 \text{ milliliters}$$

Step 2: Convert milliliters to teaspoons.

$$\frac{1 \text{ teaspoon}}{5 \text{ milliliters}} = \frac{? \text{ teaspoons}}{160 \text{ milliliters}} \rightarrow 32 \text{ teaspoons}$$

These problems cannot be solved by making a straight conversion from what is known to what is unknown. A path must be developed so that you can establish how to get the answer. Think about what conversions most closely match the problem itself, then set up the problem.

> Do not rush through the two-step conversions. These require some forethought about how to get from what is known to what is unknown.

Plastic medicine cups are used in the health care industry to measure liquid dosages. A medicine cup is typically marked off in milliliters. Often one medicine cup is 1 fluid ounce, which is 30 milliliters.

Practice

1. 1 medicine cup = _____ teaspoons

2. 3 teaspoons = _____ gtts (drops)

3. 2¼ pints = _____ ounces

4. 1 cup = _____ teaspoons

5. 1 pint = _____ tablespoons

6. 15 tablespoons = _____ cubic centimeters

7. 68,000 grams = _____ pounds

8. 28 inches = _____ millimeters

9. _____ ounces = 24 teaspoons

10. 1½ ounces = _____ teaspoons

Sometimes math problems require multiple setups. To solve these, group the work into the most logical format.

$$\frac{25\%}{1/4}$$

Example

Step 1: Look at the problem and decide what to do to make the units similar. Convert 25% into a fraction.

$$\rightarrow \frac{25}{100}$$

Step 2: Review the problem to see what operation should be completed.

$$\frac{25/100}{1/4}$$

This problem is a complex fraction. Divide the denominator of $\frac{1}{4}$ into the numerator of $\frac{25}{100}$.

$$\frac{25}{100} \div \frac{1}{4} \rightarrow \frac{25}{100} \times \frac{4}{1} = \frac{100}{100} = 1$$

Mixed Review Practice

1. $\dfrac{50\%}{1/4}$

2. $\dfrac{1:150}{1:300} \times 2$

3. $12\frac{1}{2}\% \times \dfrac{1/2}{3/4}$

4. $\dfrac{1/2\%}{4} \times 1,000$

5. $5\% \times \dfrac{1:2}{3:4}$

Converting among Systems Worksheet

Provide the following measures. Reduce to lowest terms as necessary.

	Fraction	Decimal	Ratio	Percent
1.	$\frac{7}{8}$	_____	_____	_____
2.	_____	_____	1 : 30	_____
3.	_____	_____	_____	75%
4.	$\frac{1}{17}$	_____	_____	_____
5.	_____	_____	2 : 5	_____
6.	$\frac{5}{6}$	_____	_____	_____
7.	_____	0.08	_____	_____
8.	_____	_____	_____	10.25%
9.	$\frac{3}{5}$	_____	_____	_____
10.	_____	_____	1 : 200	_____
11.	_____	1.625	_____	_____
12.	$\frac{1}{8}$	_____	_____	_____
13.	_____	_____	11 : 50	_____
14.	_____	0.15	_____	_____
15.	_____	_____	3 : 25	_____
16.	_____	0.008	_____	_____
17.	$\frac{1}{6}$	_____	_____	_____
18.	_____	_____	_____	$15\frac{1}{4}\%$
19.	_____	0.04	_____	_____

COMBINED APPLICATIONS SELF-TEST

Show all your work.

1. Convert $^3/_{75}$ to a decimal.

2. Convert $^1/_2$% to a ratio.

3. Convert 1.05 to a fraction.

4. Convert $4^1/_8$ to a ratio.

5. Convert $27^1/_4$ to a decimal.

6. Convert 12 : 200 to a percent.

7. Convert 14.25% to a ratio.

8. $3^1/_4$ cups = _____ ounces

9. 12 fluid ounces = _____ tablespoons

10. $3^1/_2$ feet = _____ centimeters

11. 18 hours = _____ minutes

12. 1 gallon = _____ cups

13. If a teaspoon has approximately 60 drops, how many drops are in $2^1/_3$ tablespoons?

14. 12% × 0.67

15. $\dfrac{15\%}{1/2}$

Unit 8

Dosage Calculations

This unit brings together the fundamental skills of the previous chapters and applies these basics to health care applications. Although new information is taught, the processes for arriving at the correct answers depend on your ability to compute using fractions, decimals, ratio, and proportion and, to a lesser degree, percents. This unit will cover the Metric System, Roman Numerals, Apothecary Measurements and Conversions, and Dosage Calculations.

This unit provides an introduction to the apothecary system and incorporates all of the math skills presented up to this point. These fundamentals will help prepare you for math applications in the health care professions.

Metric System

Metric measurements are used for many types of measurements in the health care professions. Some uses include:

- weight calculations

- dosage calculations

- grams of food intake

- height and length measurements

- measuring liquids and medications

Metric units come in base units. These units measure different types of materials.

Base Unit	Measurement Type	Examples
Liter	volume	liquids, blood, urine
Gram	weight	an item's weight an amount of medicine
Meter	length	height, length, instruments

The metric system uses units based on multiples of ten. For this reason, metric numbers are written in whole numbers or decimal numbers, never fractions. Metric conversion problems can be solved by moving the decimal either to the left or to the right. This chart resembles the decimal place value chart on page 57. Review the similarities.

Units:	kilo-	hecto-	deka	base		deci	centi-	milli-	x	x	micro
Values:	1,000	100	10	1 meter (m)		0.1	0.01	0.001			0.000001
Symbols:	k	h	da	grams (g) liter (l or L)		d	c	m			mc or μ
Mnemonic Device:	**K**iss	**h**airy	**d**ogs	**b**ut		**d**rink	**c**hocolate	**m**ilk,	m	o	**m**

Decimals and metric measurements are based on units of ten.

Using a mnemonic device helps keep the metric units in the correct sequence or order. Try something silly like "kiss hairy dogs but drink chocolate milk, mom." Knowing a device like this will help you remember the order of the units on an exam.

Note that the *mo* are placeholders. This helps one remember to count the spaces in the mnemonic device.

Using the Metric Symbols

The metric system uses the unit of measure, a prefix, and a base element to form the metric units. To form *millimeter*, take *m-* from *milli* and *m-* from *meter* and form *mm*, which represents the *millimeter*.

The metric system combines prefixes that give the unit and root words that indicate the type of measurement as in volume, weight, or length. The prefixes are the key to deciphering what number of the units you have.

Prefix	Meaning	Symbol
kilo-	thousand	k
hecto-	hundred	h
deka-	ten	da
base	one	m, g, L
deci-	tenth	d
centi-	hundredth	c

milli-	thousandth	m
micro-	millionth	mc or μ

Root	Use	Symbol
gram	weight	g
meter	length	m
liter	volume	L or l

Every metric prefix may be combined with every root. The application of these terms depends on the measurement being completed. Thus, liquids are measured in liters and dry medication uses grams because this type of drug is measured by weight.

Supply the words or abbreviations:

1. kilogram
2. ml
3. gram
4. mg
5. centimeter

6. mm
7. kilometer
8. mcg
9. L
10. kg

11. km
12. meter
13. microgram
14. kl
15. cm

> k h d b d c m m o m

You can use the first letters of the metric units to recall order by writing them on a piece of scratch paper or an answer sheet on examination days.

Changing Unit Measures

To change units within the metric system, review the number's place value and then consider where you are converting to. Count the number of spaces from the number you are starting with and the place you are converting to.

$$45.5 \text{ g} = \underline{\hspace{1cm}} \text{ mg}$$

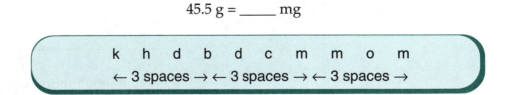

k	h	d	b	d	c	m	m	o	m
← 3 spaces →			← 3 spaces →			← 3 spaces →			

Note that the *mo* are placeholders. This helps one remember to count the spaces in the mnemonic device. Also, most conversions in health care are between the units of kilo (k), gram, meter, liter (b) and milli (m) and micro (m). There are three spaces to move between each of these to make the conversions.

From gram to milligram, there are three spaces. Note the direction from gram to milligram is to the right. Move the decimal three places to the right. Thus,

$$45.5 \text{ g} = 45500 \text{ milligrams.}$$

Note that most of the health care conversions are done between kg and g, g and mg, mg and mcg, m and cm, and L and ml. Once these are practiced, converting between units will feel natural. Practice making the conversion by moving the decimal from one unit to another. Use a pencil to draw the ∪ as you count the spaces. Start at the existing decimal and move to the right of each metric unit. Remember that "b" stands for the base units of meters, liters, or grams.

1. k h d b d c m m o m   4 g = _____ kg

2. k h d b d c m m o m   360 g = _____ mg

3. k h d b d c m m o m   9.25 kg = _____ g

4. k h d b d c m m o m   220 cc = _____ L

5. k h d b d c m m o m   _____ g = 1000 mcg

6. k h d b d c m m o m   _____ mg = 426 mcg

7. k h d b d c m m o m   _____ kg = 358.6 g

8. k h d b d c m m o m   _____ cm = 3.97 m

9. k h d b d c m m o m   37.5 mcg = _____ mg

10. k h d b d c m m o m   _____ cm = 6.75 mm

Use these letters and the mnemonic device as a quick memory tool for test recall or assignments.

In other fields, a cubic centimeter (cc) is viewed as a ▱, but in health care professions a cubic centimeter is the same as milliliter (mL or ml). The logic for this is that a syringe has a tube and measures volume in cc or ml. Thus, cc equals ml.

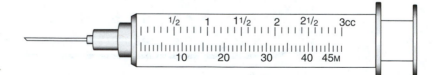

Example   Use as work space with the mnemonic device.

50 mL = _____ L   k h d b d c m, m o m

$$0.050 \underset{\cup\cup\cup}{} = 0.05L$$

Practice

1. 1cc = _____ ml

2. 0.5 L = _____ ml

3. _____ mg = 26 mcg

4. 0.75 g = _____ mg

5. 19.5 kg = _____ g

6. 15 mg = _____ g

7. _____ g = 0.3 kg

8. 8.5 L = _____ ml

9. 0.07 mg = _____ mcg

10. 4 kg = _____ mg

11. 14 cm = _____ m

12. 0.001 kg = _____ g

13. _____ L = 250 cc

14. 3.8 mg = _____ g

15. _____ mg = 0.6 g

16. 56.75 ml = _____ L

17. _____ mg = 36 g

18. _____ g = 10 mg

19. 7500 ml = _____ L

20. _____ mm = 50 cm

Units:	kilo-	hecto-	deka	base	deci	centi-	milli-	x	x	micro
Values:	1,000	100	10	1	0.1	0.01	0.001			0.000001
				meter (m)						
Symbols:	k	h	da	grams (g)	d	c		m		mc or μ
				liter (l or L)						
Mnemonic Device:	Kiss	hairy	dogs	but	drink	chocolate	milk,	m	o	m

21. 12.5 mg = _____ mcg

22. 5.78 g = _____ kg

23. 24 dm = _____ cm

24. 250 mcg = _____ mg

25. 12.76 kg = _____ g

26. 45 m = _____ mm

27. 23.5 cm = _____ mm

28. 750 µg = _____ mg

29. 800 cm = _____ m

30. 0.0975 mg = _____ mcg

31. 1,000 mL = _____ L

32. 3 kg = _____ g

33. 12,500 cm = _____ m

34. 75.5 mg = _____ mcg

35. 0.125 g = _____ mg

36. 0.150 mg = _____ mcg

37. 45,250 mg = _____ g

38. 9,500 g = _____ kg

39. 1,000 mcg = _____ g

40. 25 mcg = _____ mg

41. 5524 g = _____ kg

42. 45 mL = _____ L

43. 1.25 m _____ cm

44. 550 mcg = _____ mg

45. 0.09 L = _____ mL

46. 24.5 cm = _____ m

47. 0.1 g = _____ mg

48. 0.25 L = _____ mL

49. 8500 mcg = _____ mg

50. 0.625 g = _____ mcg

METRIC SYSTEM SELF-TEST

1. 0.75 g = _____ mg

2. _____ mg = 75 mcg

3. _____ kg = 54.6 g

4. 8.3 L = _____ cc

5. 0.014 g = _____ mcg

6. 1.2 ml = _____ L

7. 10 mcg = _____ g

8. _____ L = 250 cc

9. _____ mg = 0.015 g

10. _____ mcg = 30 mg

11. 0.008 mcg = _____ mg

12. 1.24 kg = _____ g

13. 25 cm = _____ m

14. _____ L = 2.5 mL

15. _____ cc = 65 L

Roman Numerals

In our daily lives we use Arabic numerals 0 to 9 and combinations of these digits to do most of our mathematical activities. In the health care field, Roman numerals are used along with Arabic numerals. Roman numerals are often found in prescriptions and in medical records and charts. Roman numerals consist of lower- and uppercase letters that represent numbers. For medical applications, Roman numerals will be written in lowercase, not uppercase, letters for the numbers 1 to 10. Use uppercase when smaller numbers are part of a number over 30 such as 60: LX not lx. Do not use commas in Roman numerals.

Roman Numerals

Roman numerals are formed by combining these numbers.

1 = i or I	6 = vi or VI	½ = ss
2 = ii or II	7 = vii or VII	50 = L
3 = iii or III	8 = viii or VIII	100 = C
4 = iv or IV	9 = ix or IX	500 = D
5 = v or V	10 = x or X	1,000 = M

Mnemonic Device   Note the pattern: 50-100-500-1000

L = 50	Lovely
C = 100	Cats
D = 500	Don't
M = 1000	Meow!

This will help you to remember the order and value of each Roman numeral.

Use the following basic Roman numeral concepts to accurately read and write Roman numerals.

Concept 1

Add Roman numerals of the same or decreasing value when they are placed next to each other. Read these from left to right.

Examples   vii = 5 + 2 = 7   xxi = 10 + 10 + 1 = 21

Practice   Write the numerals in Arabic or Roman numerals.

1. xiii
2. xv
3. xxxi
4. LV
5. MI

6. 17
7. 31
8. 120
9. 1½
10. 11

Concept 2

Subtract a numeral of decreasing or lesser value from the numeral to its right.

Examples   iv = 5 − 1 = 4   XC = 100 − 10 = 90

                 IM = 1000 − 1 = 999   xix = 10 + 10 − 1 = 19

Practice Write the numerals in Arabic or Roman numerals.

1. ixss   6. 19

2. XL   7. 39

3. CD   8. 24¼

4. LM   9. 240

5. XCIX   10. 499

Concept 3

When converting long Roman numerals to Arabic numerals, it is helpful to separate the Roman numerals into groups and work from both ends.

Example   CDLXXIV → CD L XX IV

1. Start with the IV = 5 − 1 = 4   4
2. Next do X + X = 20   20
3. C-D = 500 − 100 = 400   400
4. L = 50   + 50
5. Then add the elements   474

Practice 1. CXIV   6. XLss

2. LVIII   7. CDIV

3. DXIV   8. MCML

4. MDCIXss   9. DXCIIss

5. LXXXIX   10. CMLXXIVss

This method of separating the elements and working from both ends works well for converting from Arabic to Roman numerals as well.

Example Convert 637 to Roman numerals

600 DC
30 XXX
7 VII

Then rewrite the Roman numeral from the largest number on the left to the smallest numbers on the right. → DCXXXVII

Practice

1. 14½	6. 789
2. 33	7. 450
3. 146	8. 76
4. 329	9. 17
5. 999	10. 1294

Mixed Practice   Convert between Roman numerals and Arabic numerals.

1. DCCL	11. CMVIII
2. XXIVss	12. MCDLIV
3. XVIII	13. 362
4. 23	14. 16
5. 19	15. 999
6. 1,495	16. XXXIXss
7. 607	17. LXXVIII
8. CCLIVss	18. 309½
9. 66	19. 2,515
10. MVII	

20. What should you do to convert a number with decimal 0.5 in it to a Roman numeral?

Rounding in Dosage Calculations

The metric system is used to measure liquids, weights, and medicine. Rounding will make dealing with the applications more practical. To assist in this process, follow these three guidelines:

1. Any decimal that stands alone without a whole number must have a 0 placed in the whole number place. This is the standard way of noting a decimal number that does not have a whole number with it. It also helps ensure reading and interpreting the number correctly.

Examples   0.5 g   0.25 mg   0.125 mcg

2. Round decimals to the correct place value. This is somewhat dependent on your profession; however, some general guidelines exist. For example, kilogram and degrees in Celsius and Fahrenheit are placed in tenths.

3. Multi-step problems require that you convert between number systems, especially between fractions and decimals. If the drug measurement is in metrics (milligram, gram, microgram), the solution to the problem must be in decimals. There are no fractions in the metric system. Therefore, ¼ mg is stated as 0.25 mg.

> Correct formats mean correct answers!

Practice   Solve the problems below by using the three guidelines to ensure the correct format of these medications:

1. 25.89 kilograms

2. 2.7759 mL liquid medicine

3. 12.54 mg of a tablet

4. 5¼ kilograms

5. 50½ milligrams of pain medication

Apothecary Measurement and Conversions

The apothecary system is a means for calculating drug amounts for medical fields. The apothecary system relies on several number systems to denote measurements: lower case Roman numerals, Arabic numbers, and fractions. Some basic rules are applied in apothecary that do not exist in other measurement systems:

Rule 1: Fractions of ½ may be written as ss.

Rule 2: Lower case Roman numerals are used for apothecary amounts of ten or less and for the numbers 20 and 30.

Rule 3: The symbol is placed before the quantity: Thus, 7½ grains is written *grains viiss* or *gr viiss.*

In metric and household measurement, the symbol follows the quantity:

25 milligrams, 3 cups, $16^{1}/_{3}$ pounds.

Four common symbols that exist in apothecary need to be memorized:

Term	Symbol	Approximate Conversion
fluidounce	[℥]	fluid ounce 1 = drams 8
fluid dram	[ℨ]	dram 1 = 4 or 5 milliliters
minim	[♏]	
grain	gr	1 grain = 60 milligrams

Once you are familiar with these terms, symbols, and their equivalents, you will be ready to use these apothecary units in your conversions. This is a new concept for health care students to learn. We think of science and measurement as exact, but apothecary is a measurement system of approximate equivalents. Approximate equivalents come into play when you are converting among the measurement systems. Metric-to-metric or household-to-household conversions usually can be done in exact measurements. Metric- or household-to-apothecary measurement conversions generally will be done through approximate measures. The equivalents are called approximate because they are rounded to the nearest whole number. In exact measures, 1 gram is equivalent to 15.432 grains; however, the simple conversion in approximate equivalents used in health care is 1 gram = grains 15. To accomplish these conversions, you must memorize some of the approximate equivalents.

Approximate Equivalents

fluidram 1 = 1 teaspoon	1 inch = 2.5 centimeters
grain 1 = 60 milligrams	1 kilogram = 2.2 pounds
1 teaspoon = 5 milliliters	1 teaspoon = 60 drops
fluid ounce 1 = fluid drams 8	
fluid ounce 1 = 2 tablespoons	1 quart = 1 liter
fluid ounce 1 = 30 milliliters	1 cup = 250 milliliters
1 quart = fluid ounces 32	

Practice These conversions are accomplished by setting up the known and unknown in proportion format. Use the example below as your guide:

Example

$$℥ \, 2\frac{1}{2} = \underline{\quad\quad} \text{ milliliters}$$

$$\underset{known}{\underline{\quad}} \qquad \underset{unknown}{\underline{\quad}}$$

$$\frac{℥ \, 1}{30 \text{ mL}} = \frac{℥ \, 2\frac{1}{2}}{? \text{ mL}}$$

$$30 \times 2\frac{1}{2} \rightarrow 30 \times 2.5 = 75 \text{ mL}$$

Practice Conversions between metric and grains are dry equivalents. Use ratio and proportion. Show all of your work to the right of the problem.

1. 30 mg = gr _____

2. gr$^1/_4$ = _____ mg

3. 75 mg = gr _____

4. _____ mg = gr$^1/_{150}$

5. gr$^1/_6$ = _____ mg

6. gr$^1/_{100}$ = _____ mg

7. 15 g = gr _____

8. 0.8 mg = gr _____

9. gr _____ = 0.30 mg

10. 0.6 g = gr _____

11. gr iiiss = _____ mg

12. 0.05 g = gr _____

When completing multiple conversions, it is best to work within the same unit of measure before changing to another unit of measure. Do all of the metric conversions, then move to the grain conversions, or make the grain-to-metric conversion into milligrams, then convert from milligrams to grams or micrograms. By doing so, you will have only one math setup per problem. Use the standard conversion equivalents to make the conversions.

> microgram = mcg or µg

Practice

1. gr xv = _____ mg = _____ g

2. 500 mg = gr _____ = _____ g

3. 0.015 g = gr _____ = _____ mg

4. 0.0001 g = _____ mg = _____ gr

5. _____ mg = _____ mcg = gr $^1/_4$

6. 0.3 mg = gr _____ = _____ g

7. gr iss = _____ mg = _____ g

8. 400 µg = gr _____ = _____ mg

9. gr viiiss = _____ mg = _____ g

10. gr ⅛ = _____ mg

Liquid equivalents are converted in the same manner. A wider range of conversions are needed for these. Rely on the conversion charts, but work toward memorizing these equivalents so that you can efficiently apply them.
Make these liquid conversions:

Practice

1. ʒ 1 = _____ tsp

2. 15 mL = ʒ _____

3. 1 tbsp = _____ mL

4. 10 tsp = _____ mL

5. 6 tsp = ʒ _____

6. ʒ ss = _____ tsp

7. 45 ml = ʒ _____

8. 15 cc = ʒ _____

9. 20 ml = _____ tsp

10. 3 tbsp = _____ mL

11. $2\frac{1}{2}$ qt = _____ mL

12. 45 mL = ʒ _____

13. 1 tsp = _____ cc

14. $1\frac{1}{4}$ cup = _____ mL

15. 2 L = ʒ _____

16. 2 tbsp = ʒ _____

17. 15 tsp = _____ mL

18. 4 mL = _____ gtts

19. 60 mL = _____ tbsp

20. 2.5 mL = _____ tsp

Mixed Application   Make the following conversions.

1. gr $\frac{1}{2}$ = _____ mg

2. 2 tsp = _____ cc

3. $12\frac{1}{2}$ tsp = _____ cc

4. gr $\frac{1}{400}$ = _____ mg

5. $2\frac{1}{4}$ qt = _____ mL

6. 12 tsp = ʒ _____

7. ʒ 14 = _____ mL

8. 4.4 L = _____ qt

9. 35 cc = _____ tsp

10. 30 mL = ʒ _____

11. gr viii = _____ mg

12. 4 kg = _____ lbs

13. 0.3 mg = gr _____

14. $39\frac{3}{5}$ lbs = _____ kg

15. $2\frac{1}{2}$ cups = ʒ _____

16. 250 mL = _____ pint

17. ʒ 4 = _____ cup

18. 15 mL = ʒ _____

19. gr v = _____ mg

20. 120 mg = gr _____

21. gr $\frac{1}{150}$ = _____ mg

22. ʒ $\frac{1}{8}$ = ʒ _____

23. $\frac{1}{4}$ cup = ʒ _____

24. ʒ 6 = _____ mL

25. gr vii = _____ mg

26. 16 Tbsp = ℥ _____

27. ℥ 6 = _____ tbsp

28. 0.3 L = ℥ _____

29. 14 inches = _____ cm

30. 90 mg = gr _____

31. ℥ 40 = ℥ _____

32. 16 Tbsp = _____ mL

33. ℥ 3 = _____ tbsp

34. gr$^1/_{100}$ = _____ mcg

35. ℥ 64 = _____ pt

36. 0.4 mg = gr _____

37. 5 tsp = _____ cc

38. 75 mL = _____ Tbsp

39. 4$^1/_2$ cups = ℥ _____

40. 90 mL = ℥ _____

Apothecary Conversions

Notice that the conversions are set up so that the 1 elements are all on the left and that these will be placed on top of the known part of the ratio and proportion equation. This simplifies the learning process, expedites learning, and helps recall of these conversions.

Practice   Make these conversions:

1. 600 mg = gr _____

2. 180 mL = _____ tbsp

3. 24 tsp = ℥ _____

4. ℥ ss _____ tsp

5. 5 tbsp = _____ mL

6. ℥ 48 = _____ cups

7. 20 cc = _____ tsp

8. ℥ 20 = _____ cups

9. gr xv = _____ mg

10. 750 mL = _____ pints

11. 240 cc = ℥ _____

12. 0.3 mg = _____ g

13. $4^1/_2$ qt = _____ mL

14. $6^1/_2$ tsp = _____ mL

15. 0.1 mg = gr _____

16. 1500 mL = _____ cups

17. 4.5 L = _____ qt

18. ℥ 96 = _____ L

19. $1^1/_4$ cups _____ mL

20. 5 Tbsp = _____ tsp

21. ℥ iv = _____ mL

22. 500 mg = gr _____

23. 120 mL = _____ tsp

24. $2^1/_4$ cups = _____ mL

25. $3^1/_2$ cups = _____ mL

Dosage Calculations Formula

When using the dosage formula provided in this chapter, you must ensure that the medication information is in the correct place. This is true with any math formula. This formula can be used for most medication orders and is useful to memorize:

$$\frac{\text{Desired or Ordered Dosage}}{\text{Supply on Hand}} \times \text{Quantity} = \text{Unknown Dosage}$$

The formula is abbreviated as:

$$\frac{D}{H} \times Q = X$$

Note: Follow these two rules to ensure accurate setup:

Rule 1: The Dosage Ordered/Desired and the Have/Supply must be in the same unit of measure.

Rule 2: The Quantity and the Unknown Dosage will be in the same unit of measure.

Use the formula:

$$\frac{\text{Dosage (D)}}{\text{Supply on Hand (H)}} \times \text{Quantity (Q)} = \text{Medication Given}$$

The dosage is the amount of the medication that the doctor orders. The supply on hand is the available form of the drug. In other words, milligrams, grams, caplets, tablets, etc. This is what the pharmacy or the medication cabinet has on hand. The quantity is the amount of medication per tablet, milliliter, milligram, etc.

It is important the dosage and the supply on hand be in the same unit of measure. Thus, if the doctor's order is in milligrams, and you only have the medication in grams, you will convert the order to grams to match the supply that you have on hand.

You can apply this formula in two steps:

Example   The doctor orders 250 mg. The supply in the medicine cabinet is in 125 mg tablets.

$$\frac{D}{H} \times Q = X \qquad \begin{array}{l} \text{Order} = 250 \text{ mg} \\ \text{Have} = 125 \text{ mg} \end{array} \qquad \text{Quantity} = \left\{ \begin{array}{l} \text{solid form of medication,} \\ \text{and Q is 1, so the Q} \\ \text{can be eliminated as a} \\ \text{math step in this} \\ \text{problem.} \end{array} \right.$$

Step 1: Put the information into the format

$$\frac{D}{H} \times Q = X \quad \frac{250 \text{ mg}}{125 \text{ mg}}$$

Step 2: Calculate. Remember that the horizontal line indicates division, so divide 250 by 125.

The result will be 2 tablets.

Practice   1. Order: 30 mg
           Have: 10 mg per tablet
           Give: _____

    2. Order: 1 mg
           Have: 5 mg per mL
           Give: _____

    3. Order: 1500 mg
           Have: 500 mg tablets
           Give: _____

    4. Order: 15 mg
           Have: 7.5 mg per tablet
           Give: _____

5. Order: 10 mg
   Have: 20 mg per mL
   Give: _____

6. Order: 0.25 g
   Have: 50 mg per 2 mL
   Give: _____

7. Order: 1.5 mg
   Have: 3.0 mg per mL
   Give: _____

8. Order: 0.1 g
   Have: 25 mg per 2 mL
   Give: _____

9. Order: 0.15 g
   Have: 25 mg per tablet
   Give: _____

10. Order: 10 mg
    Have: 2.5 mg per capsule
    Give: _____

Now that the formula is familiar to you, the next step is to apply the metric and apothecary conversions you learned in this unit.

> Convert the unit of measure of the **order** and **have** to the same unit of measure. One guideline is that it is often easier to convert the "order" to the "have" measure unit. This also helps in being able to quickly compute the answer. Once the units are identifiable, it is easy to do.

Practice   1. Order: 1 g
              Have: 50 mg per 2 mL
              Give: _____

2. Order: 0.5 g
   Have: 200 mg per tablet
   Give: _____

3. Order: 0.15 g
   Have: 300 mg per caplet
   Give: _____

4. Order: gr x
   Have: 180 mg per mL
   Give: _____

5. Order: 0.06 g
   Have: 15 mg tablets
   Give: _____

6. Order: 1.5 g
     Have: 125 mg per 2 mL
     Give: _____

7. Order: 1.5 g
     Have: 1000 mg per tablet
     Give: _____

8. Order: gr iss
     Have: 30 mg per tablet
     Give: _____

9. Order: 1.5 g
     Have: 750 mg per tablet
     Give: _____

10. Order: gr $\frac{1}{8}$
     Have: 7.5 mg per tablet
     Give: _____

More Dosage Calculation Practice

1. Order: 25 mg po
     Have: 10 mg
     Give: _____

2. Order: 125 mg
     Have: 100 mg per 4 ml
     Give: _____

3. Order: gr iss
     Have: 50 mg per caplet
     Give: _____

4. Order: 75 mg
     Have: 25 mg per 2 mL
     Give: _____

5. Order: 25 mg po
     Have: 10 mg
     Give: _____

6. Order: 300 mg
     Have: gr v in each tablet
     Give: _____

7. Order: 12.5 mg orally after meals
     Have: 25 mg
     Give: _____

8. Order: 0.25 mg
     Have: 0.125 mg by mouth
     Give: _____

9. Order: 120 mg by mouth
   Have: gr ss per tablet
   Give: _____

10. Order: 1500 mg
    Have: 500 mg per caplet
    Give: _____

DOSAGE CALCULATIONS SELF-TEST

1. 300 mg = gr _____

2. The doctor's order is for 20 mg. Have 10 mg per 5 mL. Give _____.

3. 0.3 mg = gr _____

4. Order: 250 mg of a drug by mouth. You have scored tables in 100 mg dosages. Give _____.

5. ℥ 4 = _____ cc

6. Order: pain medication 0.6 g orally every four hours. In the supply are tablets labeled gr v of the pain medication. Give _____.

7. Order: 1.25 mg. Have 0.25 mg/5mL. Give _____.

8. Write seven and a half grains in medical notation. _____

9. The doctor orders 200 milligrams of a drug by mouth every four hours. The vial contains 125 milligrams per 5 milliliter. Give _____ mL.

10. Order: gr iii
    Have: 60 mg tablet
    Give: _____

11. Order: 50 milligrams orally
    Have: 12.5 mg in each 5 mL
    Give: _____

12. Order: gr 1/150
    Have: 200 mcg per tablet
    Give: _____

13. Order: gr v p.o.
    Have: 0.15 g per tablet
    Give: _____

14. Doctor Brown orders 0.2 grams of zidovudine in tablets every four hours for an HIV patient. The pharmacy carries this medication in 100 milligram tablets. How many tablets will the patient receive? _____

15. The nurse has 15 milligram tablets in her medicine cabinet. Doctor Smith orders 30 milligrams of Phenobarbital. She will give _____.

PRACTICE POST-TEST

Please show all your work. (Each answer is worth 2 points.)

1. The lead dental assistant spends the following amounts for supplies: $25.00 for colored pencils, $18.00 for rubber bands, $124.00 for patient folders, $129.00 for paper products, and $165.00 for rubber dams. What is the total in dollars?

2. The dental assistants switch lab jackets daily. Each dental assistant needs four jackets. If the cost per assistant is $72, how much is each jacket?

3. Dental assistants work 8 hours a day for approximately 20 days a month. About how many hours a month do they work?

4. The baby measures 26 inches at nine months of age. If the baby has grown 5 inches since birth, what was the baby's length at birth?

5. Rounding:
   a. Round 7,872 to the nearest tens _____
   b. Round 22,875 to the nearest hundreds _____

6. $\dfrac{1}{2} + \dfrac{6}{8} + \dfrac{1}{12}$

7. $\dfrac{5}{9} - \dfrac{1}{3}$

8. $3\frac{1}{4} \times 2\frac{1}{3}$

9. $200 \div \dfrac{2}{5}$

10. $65°C = \underline{\hspace{1.5cm}} °F$

11. $\dfrac{1/200}{1/4}$

12. Arrange in order from smallest to largest: 0.08, 8.88, 0.88, 8.08, 1.08

13. Rounding:
   a. Round 10.295 to the nearest tenth   _____
   b. Round 0.0586 to the nearest hundredth   _____

14. 25 + 0.125 + 2.27

15. 4.6 − 0.68

16. 25.4 × 2.5

17. 32.04 ÷ 0.08

18. 93.23 × 100

19. Conversions:

    a. Convert 0.08 to a fraction   _____

    b. Convert $^7/_8$ to a decimal   _____

20. 1.2 × $^1/_{25}$. Write your answer as a fraction.

21. Metric conversion:

    a. 25.75 g = _____ mg

    b. 325 mcg = _____ mg

        c. _____ kg = 5,575 g

        d. 2 L = _____ cc

        e. 35 mm = _____ cm

22. $4 : 8\frac{1}{4} = x : 5.5$

23. $\frac{1}{300} : \frac{1}{125} = x : 1$

24. What is 45% of 424?

25. $\frac{1}{4}$% of 600 is _____

26. There are _____ grams of pure drug in a 55% solution.

27. The net cost of an instrument listed at $3,356.50 with a single trade discount of 20% is _____.

28. Express 2 : 20 as a percent

29. **a.** Express $^{1}/_{2}$% as a fraction

    b. Express 15 : 90 as a decimal

    c. Express $0.65^{1}/_{4}$ as a percent

    d. Express 55% as a ratio

30. 2500 mL = _____ pints

31. 64 cm = _____ inches

32. Write the Roman numerals:

    a. $8^{1}/_{2}$ _____

    b. 155 _____

33. Make the apothecary conversions:

    a. 0.6 mg = gr _____

    b. gr $^{1}/_{150}$ = _____ g

    c. $12^{1}/_{2}$ tsp = _____ mL

    d. 32 fluid ounces = _____ cups

    e. 25 mL = _____ tsp

34. Solve:

    a. Order: 0.125 g
       Have: 100 g per 5 mL
       Give: _____

    b. Order: gr v
       Have: 300 mg per 2 cc
       Give: _____

Answer Key

Unit 2

a. 1,023

b. 71,371

c. 9,246

d. 750

e. 105 R 75 or 105.3 or $105^{3}/_{10}$

f. 2,390, 4,500

g. 308

Unit 3

a. $9^{17}/_{24}$

b. $4^{13}/_{16}$

c. $48^{1}/_{3}$

d. 640

e. $5^{15}/_{52}$

f. $1^{1}/_{5}$

g. 6

Unit 4

a. 17.9, 17.58, 17.059

b. 83.3 F, $14.11

c. 14.4 C, 100.4 F

d. 0.009, 0.125, 0.1909, 0.25, 0.3

e. 15.87

f. 769.2

g. $108.90 for 30 or the pack of 30

h. 78

Unit 5

a. varies: $\dfrac{2}{8}, \dfrac{3}{12}, \dfrac{4}{16}$, or 2 : 8, 3 : 12, or 4 : 16, etc.

b. 120

c. 22.67 or $22^{2}/_{3}$

d. $\dfrac{1}{2}$

e. 90

Unit 6

a. 30

b. 136.5

Unit 7

a.

Fractions	Decimals	Ratio	Percent
$2/5$	0.4	2 5	40%
$17/100$	0.17	17 : 100	17%
$27/50$	0.54	27 : 50	54%
$1/5$	0.2	1 : 5	20%

b. Standard measurement and metric conversions:

2 tablespoons = 6 teaspoons

8 pints = 4 quarts

16 ounces = 2 cups

1 fluid ounce = 2 tablespoon(s)

23.5 kilograms = 51.7 pounds

c. 280 milligrams, 25.3 grams, 111 calories

d. $\frac{2}{3}$

e. 3.5

f. $\frac{3}{5}$

g. $\frac{7}{200}$ or 0.035

Unit 8

a. 1850 mg, 560 mcg, 230 cm, 13625 g, 1000 mL

b. 18, CIX, 549, LXIV, $6\frac{1}{2}$

c. 45, $\frac{1}{100}$, 16, 45, 6

d. $\frac{1}{2}$ tab, 1 tab, $\frac{1}{2}$ tab, 2.5 mL, 2 caps

Unit 2: Whole Number Review

Addition Practice: pp. 10–11

1. 19
3. 492
5. 2,063
7. 488
9. 2,664

Addition Applications: p. 11

1. a. 266
   b. 711
   c. 1,176
   d. 20 boxes
3. a. 300
   b. 720
   c. 75
   d. 110
   e. 1,205

Subtraction Practice: p. 12

1. 394
3. 235
5. 437

7. 1,873
9. 4,212

Subtraction Applications: pp. 12–13

1. 1,474
3. 3 boxes

Multiplication Practice: p. 14

1. 96
3. 23,508
5. 99,960
7. 12,288
9. 92,656
11. 4,152

Multiplication Applications: p. 14

1. $3,444.00
3. $525.00

Division Setup Practice: p. 15

1. $76\overline{)145}$
3. $17\overline{)49}$
5. $8\overline{)2,044}$

Division Practice: p. 17

1. 94
3. 3,086 R 1
5. 311
7. 1,576 R 8
9. 23,441
11. 12,506 R 1

Division Applications: pp. 17–18

1. 13 days
3. $21
5. $1,656.00
7. 9 grams

Rounding Practice: p. 19

1. a. 3,920
   b. 140

c. 6,950

d. 1,930

e. 15,930

f. 100

3. a. 3,000

b. 88,000

c. 7,000

d. 13,000

e. 433,000

f. 3,000

Estimation Practice: p. 19

1. a. $194

b. $162

c. $112

d. $2,914

Average Practice: pp. 20–21

1. $9

3. 5

Whole Number Self-Test: pp. 21–23

1. 1,621

3. 7 dollars

5. 16

7. 17

9. $966.00

11. 110

13. ten thousands

14. 8,910

15. 31,400

Unit 3: Fractions

Part to Whole Relationships: p. 25

1. Three parts to four total parts

3. Seven parts to eight total parts

Equivalent Fractions Practice: p. 26

1. 6

3. 8

5. 15

7. 36

9. 54

Reducing Fractions Practice: pp. 27–28

1. $\frac{1}{7}$

3. $\frac{1}{2}$

5. $\frac{1}{4}$

7. $\frac{1}{2}$

9. $\frac{1}{3}$

Reducing Mixed Numbers Practice: p. 28

1. $13\frac{1}{4}$

3. $1\frac{1}{2}$

5. $3\frac{1}{4}$

7. $2\frac{1}{9}$

9. $6\frac{1}{2}$

Fractional Parts from Words Practice: p. 29

1. $\frac{2}{5}$

3. $\frac{1}{3}$

5. $\frac{1}{8}$

Improper Fractions to Mixed Numbers Practice: pp. 29–30

1. $7\frac{1}{2}$

3. $19\frac{1}{2}$

5. $9\frac{3}{7}$

7. $2\frac{3}{8}$

9. 1

Adding Like Denominators
Practice: pp. 31–32

1. 1

3. 2

5. $\dfrac{7}{12}$

7. $\dfrac{7}{13}$

9. $22\frac{5}{6}$

11. $\dfrac{4}{5}$

13. 1

15. $140\frac{1}{4}$

Finding Common Denominator
Practice: pp. 32–33

1. 20

3. 44

5. 25

7. 200

9. 27

Adding Unlike Fractions
Practice: pp. 33–34

1. $\dfrac{17}{20}$

3. $1\frac{1}{9}$

5. $\dfrac{1}{2}$

7. $\dfrac{13}{21}$

9. $1\frac{1}{15}$

11. $1\frac{2}{5}$

13. $106\frac{8}{9}$

15. $8\frac{7}{8}$

Finding the Common Denominator
Practice: p. 35

1. 20

3. 192

5. 45

7. 36

9. 30

Adding Fractions Practice: pp. 35–36

1. $9\frac{11}{12}$

3. $13\frac{1}{2}$

5. $6\frac{5}{7}$

7. $18\frac{29}{30}$

9. $18\frac{9}{10}$

11. $16\frac{17}{27}$

13. $39\frac{5}{12}$

15. $13\frac{7}{15}$

17. $4\frac{7}{16}$

19. $5\frac{1}{2}$

Addition Applications: p. 36

1. $121\frac{3}{4}$

3. $1\frac{3}{16}$

5. $3\frac{5}{6}$

Ordering Fractions Practice: p. 37

1. $\dfrac{4}{12}, \dfrac{1}{4}, \dfrac{2}{9}$

3. $\dfrac{20}{50}, \dfrac{33}{100}, \dfrac{6}{25}$

Subtracting Like Fractions Practice: p. 38

1. $\dfrac{1}{9}$

3. $\dfrac{2}{11}$

5. $2\frac{1}{6}$

7. $45\frac{1}{8}$

9. $\dfrac{1}{2}$

11. $\dfrac{1}{4}$

13. $12\frac{1}{5}$

15. $31\frac{1}{9}$

17. $124\frac{1}{12}$

19. $12\frac{5}{33}$

Subtracting Mixed Numbers from Whole Numbers Practice: p. 40

1. $10\frac{1}{6}$
3. $9\frac{3}{4}$
5. $14\frac{6}{13}$
7. $5\frac{6}{7}$
9. $10\frac{2}{5}$

Subtracting Fractions Practice: pp. 40–41

1. $7\frac{13}{20}$
3. $19\frac{17}{30}$
5. $5\frac{17}{22}$
7. $111\frac{23}{30}$
9. $31\frac{5}{8}$
11. $16\frac{5}{6}$
13. $76\frac{25}{36}$
15. $6\frac{1}{2}$

Subtraction Application: p. 41

1. $11\frac{1}{2}$
3. $99\frac{1}{4}$
5. $3\frac{1}{2}$

Multiplication Practice: pp. 41–42

1. $\frac{1}{16}$
3. $\frac{28}{45}$
5. $\frac{3}{35}$
7. $\frac{4}{9}$
9. $\frac{13}{66}$

Multiplication: Fractions and Whole Numbers Practice: p. 43

1. $1\frac{1}{2}$
3. $16\frac{1}{3}$
5. $5\frac{3}{5}$

7. $11\frac{2}{3}$
9. 4

Multiplication Practice: pp. 44–45

1. $1\frac{5}{7}$
3. $\frac{1}{4}$
5. $\frac{1}{20}$
7. $\frac{1}{4}$
9. $\frac{11}{96}$

Making Improper Fractions Practice: pp. 45–46

1. $\frac{33}{4}$
3. $\frac{88}{5}$
5. $\frac{27}{12}$
7. $\frac{32}{9}$
9. $\frac{53}{12}$

Multiplying Fractions: p. 47

1. $\frac{29}{84}$
3. $\frac{21}{40}$
5. $\frac{20}{27}$
7. $40\frac{1}{4}$
9. $3\frac{17}{20}$

Multiplication Application: pp. 47–48

1. 70 doses
3. 875 milligrams
5. $18\frac{3}{4}$ cups

Dividing Fractions Practice: pp. 49–50

1. $\frac{5}{7}$

3. $\frac{7}{24}$

5. 8

7. $\frac{1}{45}$

9. $\frac{1}{120}$

11. $3\frac{8}{9}$

13. $2\frac{7}{9}$

15. $4\frac{8}{9}$

17. $\frac{31}{130}$

19. $1\frac{47}{105}$

Division Applications: p. 50

1. $9\frac{3}{20}$

3. $13.30

5. 10

Celsius to Fahrenheit Temperature Conversions Practice: p. 51

1. 68

3. 77

5. 104

7. 176

Fahrenheit to Celsius Temperature Conversions Practice: p. 52

1. 40

3. 10

5. 15

7. 30

Complex Fractions Practice: p. 53

1. $\frac{3}{32}$

3. $\frac{1}{15,000}$

5. $1\frac{1}{5}$

7. $\frac{4}{5}$

9. $\frac{15}{16}$

Mixed Complex Fraction Problems Practice: p. 54

1. 5

3. 12

Fraction Self-Test: pp. 54–55

1. $\frac{1}{4}$

3. $11\frac{1}{11}$

5. $39\frac{4}{5}$

7. $\frac{4}{9}$

9. $\frac{2}{12}, \frac{1}{4}, \frac{1}{3}, \frac{3}{8}$

11. more

13. 5/8

15. 26 5/24

Unit 4: Decimals

Decimals in Words: pp. 57–58

1. Seven tenths

3. Five hundredths

5. One hundred fifty and seventy-five thousandths

7. One hundred twenty-five and twenty-three thousandths

9. Eighteen and eight hundredths

Words to Decimals: p. 58

1. 0.2

3. 300.002

5. 6.03

Rounding to the Nearest Tenth Practice: p. 59

1. 6.7
3. 0.8
5. 25.0 or 25
7. 0.1
9. 9.9

Rounding to the Nearest Hundredth Practice: p. 59

1. 17.33
3. 4.82
5. 0.01
7. 32.65
9. 46.09

Smaller Decimals Practice: p. 60

1. 0.89
3. 2.012
5. 0.0033

Larger Decimals Practice: p. 60

1. 0.0785
3. 0.5
5. 0.675

Ordering from Largest to Smallest Practice: p. 61

1. 7.5, 7.075, 0.75, 0.7, 0.07
3. 5.55, 5.15, 5.05, 0.5, 0.05

Adding Decimals Practice: pp. 61–62

1. 38.15
3. 86.235
5. 89.2496
7. 127.52
9. 214.281

Addition Applications: p. 62

1. 4.5 milligrams
3. 226 milligrams
5. 124.54 centimeters

Subtracting Decimals Practice: p. 63

1. 0.72
3. 14.065
5. 3.5013
7. 0.175
9. 87.436

Subtraction Applications: pp. 63–64

1. 0.65 liters
3. 1.5 milligrams
5. 1.8°F

Multiplying Decimals Practice: pp. 65–66

1. 12.6
3. 33.6
5. 128.38
7. 0.8088
9. 0.4726
11. 0.0024
13. 151.11
15. 1.65036
17. 7.632
19. 6,942.53
21. 1,342.11
23. 10.04565

Multiplication Applications: p. 66

1. $420.80
3. $1,618.20
5. $128.00

Dividing Decimals Practice: pp. 67–68

1. 0.63
3. 0.232
5. 0.12

7. 52.4

9. 3.02

Dividing with Zeros as Placeholders Practice: p. 68

1. 1,060

3. 2.08

5. 1.099

7. 30.66

9. 0.2099

Simplified Multiplication Practice: pp. 69–70

1. 135

3. 1,257.5

5. 6

7. 12,670

9. 476

11. 13.45

13. 10.09

15. 23,850

Simplified Division Practice: pp. 70–71

1. 1.29

3. 12.5

5. 0.025

7. 0.158

9. 0.325

11. 10.01

13. 0.03076

15. 0.10275

Division Applications: p. 71

1. $63.25

3. 3 tablets

5. $26.24

Decimal to Fraction Conversion Practice: pp. 72–73

1. $\frac{1}{25}$

3. $6\frac{1}{4}$

5. $225\frac{1}{20}$

7. $7\frac{3}{4}$

9. $9\frac{3}{10}$

Fraction to Decimal Conversion Practice: p. 74

1. 0.5

3. 0.875

5. 0.24

7. 0.2

9. $0.83\frac{1}{3}$ or $0.08\overline{3}$

Temperature Conversions with Decimals Practice: pp. 75–76

1. 93.2

3. 224.6

5. 107.6

7. 38

9. 53.6

Mixed Fraction and Decimal Problems Practice: p. 77

1. 2.2

3. 7.5

5. 0.168

7. 7.675

Decimal Self-Test: pp. 78–79

1. Forty-five thousandths

3. 16.925

5. 90.2

7. 8.018, 0.81, 0.08, 0.018

9. 2 milligrams

11. 1/8

13. 3.625

15. 1.7

Unit 5: Ratio and Proportion

Ratios: p. 81

1. 5 : 7

3. 1 : 5

5. 1 : 2

Proportions: p. 81

1. No
3. Yes
5. No

Solving with Proportions Practice: p. 82

1. 7.5
3. 16
5. 27
7. 14
9. 52

Measurement Conversions Using Proportions Practice: pp. 84–85

1. $7\frac{2}{3}$
3. 8
5. 9
7. 4
9. 56
11. $2\frac{1}{2}$
13. 5
15. $1\frac{1}{2}$
17. 80
19. 5

Word Problems Using Proportions Practice: p. 86

1. 3 caplets
3. 17.5 grams
5. 28 kilograms

Solving for x in Complex Problems Practice: p. 88

1. 6
3. 9.6
5. 1
7. $1\frac{1}{3}$
9. 2.4
11. 1.5

Nutrition Applications: p. 89

1. 9
3. 9
5. 48
7. 1312

Other Uses for Proportions: pp. 89–90

1. 645
3. 220
5. 121.5

Ratio and Proportion Self-Test: pp. 90–91

1. Answers vary.
3. 9
5. 125
7. 8 tablets
9. $\frac{1}{75}$
11. 2 minutes 10 seconds
13. 640
15. 96 ounces

Unit 6: Percents

Percent-to-Decimal Practice: p. 94

1. 0.45
3. $0.78\frac{1}{5}$ or 0.782
5. $0.44\frac{1}{2}$ or 0.445

Decimal-to-Percent Practice: p. 94

1. 62.5%
3. 860%
5. 7.6%

Mixed Practice: p. 95

1. 0.7689
3. 0.86
5. 7.8%
7. $125\frac{1}{4}\%$ or 125.25%
9. 0.015

Setup of Percents Practice: p. 96

1. $\dfrac{25}{100} = \dfrac{x}{200}$

3. $\dfrac{8.5}{100} = \dfrac{x}{224}$

5. $\dfrac{x}{100} = \dfrac{18}{150}$

7. $\dfrac{x}{100} = \dfrac{75}{90}$

9. $\dfrac{50}{100} = \dfrac{75}{x}$

Percents Practice: p. 96–97

1. 18.
3. 25%
5. 5.88
7. 22.5%
9. 17.60

More Complex Percents Practice: p. 98

1. 41.67
3. 60
5. 15.63
7. 1280
9. 533.33

Percent Strength Practice: p. 99

1. 1 gram of pure drug to 25 mL of solution
3. 1.5 grams of pure drug to 100 mL of solution
5. 1 gram of pure drug to 20 mL of solution

Percent Equivalents in Solutions Practice: pp. 100–101

1. a. 1.25 g
   b. 1.75 g
   c. 3.25 g
   d. 6.25 g
3. a. 30%
   b. 60 g

Single Trade Discounts Practice: p. 101

1. $71.33 $404.17
3. $15.69 $109.86
5. $88.23 $264.67
7. $112.68 $137.72
9. $63.20 $94.80

Percent Self-Test: pp. 103–104

1. Answers vary. A percent is a number which is part of a whole. 75% is 75 parts of 100.
3. 243.75
5. 200
7. 2.25 grams of pure drug
9. 8.3% or 8 1/3%
11. 12%
13. 6.4%
15. 70,000

Unit 7: Combined Applications

Conversions: pp. 108–109

	Fraction	Decimal	Ratio	Percent
1.	$3/4$	0.75	3 : 4	75%
3.	$1/2$	0.5	1 : 2	50%
5.	$1/250$	0.004	1 : 250	0.4%
7.	$3/50$	0.06	3 : 50	6%
9.	$1/10$	0.1	1 : 10	10%
11.	$1\tfrac{9}{25}$	1.36	34 : 25	136%
13.	$2/5$	0.4	2 : 5	40%
15.	$16/25$	0.64	16 : 25	64%
17.	$5/6$	$0.83\tfrac{1}{3}$	5 : 6	$83\tfrac{1}{3}\%$
19.	$1/100$	0.01	1 : 100	1%

Using Combined Applications in measurement conversion Abbreviations: p. 109

1. Foot
3. Ounce
5. Pound

7. Quart

9. Drop

Standard Units of Measurement Conversion Review: pp. 110–111

1. $2\frac{1}{2}$

3. 31.25 or 31.75

5. 3

7. 24

9. $2\frac{1}{2}$

More Combined Applications Practice: p. 112

1. 6

3. 36

5. 32

7. 149.6

9. 4

Mixed Review Practice: pp. 112–113

1. 2

3. $\frac{1}{12}$

5. $\frac{1}{30}$

Converting among Systems: p. 113

	Fraction	Decimal	Ratio	Percent
1.	$\frac{7}{8}$	0.875	7 : 8	$87\frac{1}{2}\%$
3.	$\frac{3}{4}$	0.75	3 : 4	75%
5.	$\frac{2}{5}$	0.40	2 : 5	40%
7.	$\frac{2}{25}$	0.08	2 : 25	8%
9.	$\frac{3}{5}$	0.6	3 : 5	60%
11.	$1\frac{5}{8}$	1.625	13 : 8	162.5%
13.	$\frac{11}{50}$	0.22	11 : 50	22%
15.	$\frac{3}{25}$	0.12	3 : 25	12%
17.	$\frac{1}{6}$	$0.16\frac{2}{3}$	1 : 6	$16\frac{2}{3}\%$
19.	$\frac{1}{25}$	0.04	1 : 25	4%

Combined Application Self-Test: p. 114

1. 0.04

3. $1\frac{1}{20}$

5. 27.25

7. 57 : 400

9. 24

11. 1,080

13. 420

15. 0.3

Unit 8: Dosage Calculations

Units Practice: p. 117

1. kg

3. g

5. cm

7. km

9. liter

11. kilometer

13. mcg or μg

15. centimeter

Metric Conversions: p. 118

1. 0.004

3. 9,250

5. 0.001

7. 0.3586

9. 0.0375

Conversion Practice: pp. 119–121

1. 1

3. 0.026

5. 19,500

7. 300

9. 70

11. 0.14

13. 0.25

15. 600

17. 36,000

19. 7.5

21. 12,500

23. 240

25. 12,760

27. 235

29. 8

31. 1

33. 125

35. 125

37. 45.25

39. 0.001

41. 5.524

43. 125

45. 90

47. 100

49. 8.5

Metric Self-Test: p. 121

1. 750

3. 0.0546

5. 14,000

7. 0.00001

9. 15

11. 0.000008 mg

13. 0.25 m

15. 65000 cc

Roman Numerals: Concept 1 Practice: p. 122

1. 13

3. 31

5. 1001

7. xxxi

9. iss

Concept 2 Practice: p. 123

1. $9\frac{1}{2}$

3. 400

5. 99

7. xxxix

9. CCXL

Concept 3 Practice: p. 123

1. 114

3. 514

5. 89

7. 404

9. $592\frac{1}{2}$

Practice: p. 124

1. xivss

3. CXLVI

5. IM

7. CDL

9. xvii

Mixed Practice: p. 124

1. 750

3. 18

5. xix

7. DCVII

9. LXVI

11. 908

13. CCCLXII

15. IM

17. 78

19. MMDXV

Rounding in Dosage Calculations Practice: p. 125

1. 25.9

3. 12.5

5. 50.5

Apothecary Conversions Practice: p. 127

1. ss

3. $1\frac{1}{4}$

5. 10

7. 250

9. $\frac{1}{200}$

11. 210

Apothecary Equivalents Practice: p. 127

1. 900, 0.9
3. $\frac{1}{4}$, 15
5. 15, 15,000
7. 90, 0.09
9. 510, 0.51

Liquid Apothecary Equivalents Practice: p. 128

1. 6
3. 15
5. 1
7. iss
9. 4
11. 2,500
13. 5
15. 64
17. 75
19. 4

Mixed Apothecary Applications: pp. 128–129

1. 30
3. 62.5
5. 2,250
7. 420
9. 7
11. 480
13. $\frac{1}{200}$
15. 20
17. $\frac{1}{2}$
19. 300
21. 0.4
23. ii

25. 420
27. 12
29. 35 or 35.56
31. v
33. 6
35. 4
37. 25
39. 36

Apothecary Conversions Practice: pp. 129–130

1. x
3. 4
5. 75
7. 4
9. 900
11. 8
13. 4,500
15. $\frac{1}{600}$
17. $4\frac{1}{2}$
19. 312.5
21. 120
23. 24
25. 875

Dosage Calculations Practice: pp. 131–132

1. 3 tablets
3. 3 tablets
5. 0.5 mL
7. 0.5 mL
9. 6 tablets

Two-step Dosage Calculations Practice: pp. 132–133

1. 40 mL
3. $\frac{1}{2}$ caplet
5. 4 tablets

7. $1\frac{1}{2}$ tablets

9. 2 tablets

Dosage Calculation Practice: pp. 133–134

1. 2.5 mg

3. 2 caps

5. 2.5 tabs

7. $\frac{1}{2}$ tab

9. 4 tabs

Dosage Calculations
Self-Test: pp. 134–135

1. gr v

3. gr $\frac{1}{200}$

5. 120 cc

7. Give 5 mL

9. 8 mL, 3 ii

11. 20 mL

13. 2 tablets

15. 2 tablets

Practice Post-Test: pp. 136–140

1. $461.00

3. 160

5. a. 7,870

   b. 22,900

7. $\frac{2}{9}$

9. 500

11. $\frac{1}{50}$

13. a. 10.3

    b. 0.06

15. 3.92

17. 400.5

19. a. $\frac{2}{25}$

    b. 0.875

21. a. 25,750

    b. 0.325

    c. 5.575

    d. 2,000

    e. 3.5

23. $\frac{5}{12}$

25. 1.5

27. $2,685.20

29. a. $\frac{1}{200}$

    b. 0.16? or 0.167

    c. $65\frac{1}{4}$% or 65.25%

    d. 11:20

31. 25.6 or $25\frac{3}{5}$

33. a. $\frac{1}{100}$

    b. 0.4 mg

    c. 62.5 mL

    d. 4

    e. 5

Index